Dance and Belonging

Dance and Belonging

Implicit Bias and Inclusion in Dance Education

Crystal U. Davis

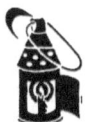

McFarland & Company, Inc., Publishers
Jefferson, North Carolina

This book has undergone peer review.

ISBN (print) 978-1-4766-8445-1
ISBN (ebook) 978-1-4766-4789-0

LIBRARY OF CONGRESS AND BRITISH LIBRARY
CATALOGUING DATA ARE AVAILABLE

Library of Congress Control Number 2022038727

© 2022 Crystal U. Davis. All rights reserved

No part of this book may be reproduced or transmitted in any form or by any means, electronic or mechanical, including photocopying or recording, or by any information storage and retrieval system, without permission in writing from the publisher.

Front cover image © T-Design/Shutterstock

Printed in the United States of America

*McFarland & Company, Inc., Publishers
Box 611, Jefferson, North Carolina 28640
www.mcfarlandpub.com*

Table of Contents

Preface	1
Introduction: Biases and Behavior	9
1. Privilege, Power, and Positionality: The Myth of Equality	31
2. Social Markers of Bias	51
3. Dance Aesthetics: A Site for Bias	65
4. Biases and Behaviors: Manifestations of Bias	78
5. Feeders and Disruptors of Bias	114
6. Numbers, Qualities, and Bodies: Solutions for Implicit Bias	136
7. Reintegration: A Fuller Picture	171
Appendix A: Social Justice Curriculum Design Outline	193
Appendix B: Community Norms Sample	194
Chapter Notes	195
Works Cited	207
Index	215

Preface

This book is about how implicit bias manifests itself in the field of dance education. The topic of implicit bias came from a lifetime of feeling like an outsider in a number of arenas inside the dance world. In dance, so many of the assumptions I was surrounded by in my dance training and creative research endeavors felt both familiar to me yet not quite part of who I was. Even as an adult in professional settings, the signals of my outsider status were so complex, I often would vent that I was unsure of whether sentiment in each case of feeling marginalized was based on my race as a Black person, my gender as a woman, or my professional expertise as a dancer. These identity markers all have some level of alienation in the context of the dominant values within the U.S. educational and performing arts settings. Things would take place such as awkward pauses and stares at me in discussions about hairstyles for performances, diminishing or completely ignoring comments I shared in education or dance production meetings as if I were not present, or high school counselors advising students not to take my dance classes to strengthen the rigor of their college applications.

The particular effects of racial bias in my dance education experiences are potent and thus provide a larger number of illustrations of implicit bias throughout this book. While race often feels rather significant for me, I thought it important to address the broader conversation of the ways that a person's visual markers of identity trigger negative effects of implicit bias in dance settings. For this reason, I discuss a variety of facets of implicit bias, not just implicit racial bias, in this book, though in my personal lived experience, race is often most influential.

In the dance studio, I found a measure of release from this lack of belonging no matter the form of dance I was learning. There was power, agency, and expression in dance that affirmed a space for my moving body in the world even if the messages about if or where I belonged in the field of dance did not fully affirm that sense of belonging. I started out learning ballet with dreams of graduating into pointe work. At my local studio the two-year-old ballet class also included tap. After a year or two of taking the combination ballet and tap class, the studio class structure in the four- or five-year-old classes added jazz to the class structure. As dance students at the studio got older, the genres then broke apart to become separate classes. Students could choose to deepen study in one of the three forms. I continued taking ballet, tap, and jazz into my teen years. In high school, I was introduced to modern dance by way of a summer camp taught by dance teachers from the North Carolina School of the Arts. The wild abandon I felt shifting weight and using momentum was unlike anything I had felt in the other forms. I was immediately hooked. In college I continued studying modern dance and was introduced to postmodern dance and somatics. The idea of disrupting norms, questioning cultural assumptions about what *dance* and *performance* meant, and moving with a full attention to body-mind as a whole and integrated source of knowledge resonated with me. By way of foremothers like Yvonne Rainer, Blondell Cummings, Irmgard Bartenieff, and Peggy Hackney, I felt like I found my creative home, my dance community. My aesthetic and creative research identity is still linked to these lineages.

While my love for dance blossomed at an early age, and I never stopped dancing, I still have moments of feeling like an outsider in some dance spaces. As an African American girl growing up in a predominantly African American North Carolina town run by mostly White people, I often felt like an outsider in my extra-curricular classes whether horseback riding or competition dance classes. The discomfort of feeling like an outsider made my discovery of dance ethnography in college a natural fit. As I navigated socially unfamiliar environments, I also learned about dances and cultures that were unfamiliar to me. In turn, my appreciation for my own culture, those daily practices, sayings, foods, and family histories, grew deeper as I began to understand how it was different from other cultures. In my undergraduate senior year of college, I merged my comparative religion major with a minor in dance and studied the relationship between religious beliefs and dance via dance ethnography research in Jodhpur, India. My studies soon led me to a profound discovery: So much of what I regarded as cultural norms were not "norms" at all. Further, the fact that these norms weren't even really *mine* to begin with has been a place that reframed much of my relationship with dance after that pivotal experience. Sure, they were the norms of where I grew up, but they were not of my own creation. Rather these norms were a matter of what I was exposed to while growing up. What I thought were my beliefs and understanding of the world were really pre-established messages that family, friends, teachers, and community members have shared with me through language/word, behaviors/deed, image/media content, and value statements. Things such as the idea that "children are to be seen and not heard"; "sitting on the ground is unclean"; "wearing shoes around the house is an acceptable level of cleanliness"; and "ballet is the foundation of all dance forms." Assumptions I previously neglected to question while living in the United States were upended through pedestrian movement and daily exchanges with people in Jodhpur, India. As a result of these conceptual seeds, my understanding of dance and dance education evolved into decades of study through two graduate degrees and continued exploration in my current research.

One example of how these ideas showed up in my dance scholarship and creative work relates to my choreographic process. My perspective on the world and dance stemmed from my religious background as a Black Southern Baptist Christian woman, socialized in the U.S., and from my training as a dancer. The monotheistic, male divinity—who I was used to encountering with either no visual representation or as a White man—was no longer the center of religious practice in Indian temples. Everywhere I traveled in Jodhpur, there were goddesses and divine presences in every aspect of daily life. They included naturally occurring symbols of deities such as rivers and stones, as well as physical representations of deities in temples.

The pantheon of expressions of divinity I experienced in India affected my creative possibilities in making dances. Instead of thinking of a single correct choreographic solution or one expression of divine perfection, the multitude of divine expressions I saw in India resulted in more freedom creatively in my dance work. This exposure to a different sensibility of creative expression changed how I approached my choreographic process. My approach shifted from a methodical process of operational thinking to a playful, celebratory exploration of infinite possibilities. Exposure to ideas about the divine Good being a myriad of expressions resulted in a more robust choreographic approach to my dance works.

My identity as an African American woman perplexed many people in India. I was the color of many South Indians. Many could not sort out other aspects of my person, such as my *oddly* coiled hair. Yet, my previous experiences deciphering cultural situations as African Americans often do in the United States, often for our own safety, meant that I could listen and learn about the interpersonal dynamics of power with a different lens than my fellow travelers, who were predominantly White. My White-bodied[1] classmates began to express their novel frustration of being treated differently and in accordance with the stereotypes that preceded them on the trip via U.S. media content. I relished my classmates having a newfound, common lived experience that I could relate to even if it were only applicable for them during the months we were in India.

My dance experiences in India differed from my ballet, tap, jazz, modern, and postmodern dance training in the United States. In India, dance classes were traditionally taught with the dance instructor sitting for most of the session, while the students danced to the teacher's verbal and rhythmic cues. It was a new form of learning dance for me. This pedagogical approach required two things. One is a rather intimate sense of the vocabulary of the dance form with little to no demonstration during the class session. The second requirement that felt new for me, is physical agency to embody a movement language not based on mimicry of a physical form moving through the steps along with me. It meant a fuller investment in each movement choice as I went through movement phrases and a clearer delineation of what I knew or didn't know in the movement phrase. So many years in my own dance training I had simply followed along while watching my dance teacher with little memory retention or awareness of how I was moving while I simulated what I was seeing. This new method of learning dance required a more active memory retention and recall as well as a more dedicated attention to making choices on how to execute the steps as accurately as possible.

I carried this new kind of dance instruction I had experienced in Jodhpur into my creative practice as a dancer, as well as my research. This new perspective of so many ways of being, seeing, and understanding the world traveled back with me to the U.S., affecting what felt like every exchange I had with people. Essentially, my perception of "standard" and "true" was called into question. For example, I knew from personal experience that ballet as the foundation of all dance forms was not only untrue but only a plausible argument in select areas on the planet. Previously, through my academic research and my teaching, I typically focused on the failures and missed moments in any learning experience as a site to fix or eliminate the errors. After my time in India, I realized that these moments of failure represented the richest sites for learning in the dance studio. For example, my inability to access the ankle flexion I aspired to in the classical Indian dance form Kucchipudi may have had as much to do with my mother's gait modeling and ballet training encouraging me to walk with my weight in the balls of my feet with my heels never touching the floor while walking. Moments of disconnect and confusion were not failures, but gleeful opportunities to learn something new—both about myself and, more importantly, about my students, colleagues, and friends. The disarray of foundational perceptions—i.e., as a dance teacher you stand at the front of the class and model movement while students follow along—was fertile ground I would now plow. I questioned the roots of long-held beliefs, while pruning the parts of those elements of my socialization that no longer held true for me. My habitual impulse to make assumptions about my students, many of whom I now realized I had little cultural context to understand, slowed.

These intersections between my own experiences and those of others engender joy for me. It is the site where my own reading, questioning, and experiences interface with unimaginably complex experiences of other people's identities and backgrounds. It is exhilarating, learning about people, how they understand the world, and how best to teach, collaborate with, and learn from each individual. I am inspired when I discover moments where I ask myself, "Why did I assume my understanding about this was the most obvious?" It is gratifying to forge a deeper connection with those who have a different sense of dance and dance education. In these moments we get to see each other more fully as our distinct selves.

Even as I write this book, assumptions and perspectives are being disrupted and questioned. The Covid-19 pandemic has displaced me from conducting embodied in-person work around racism and dance. I could no longer conduct in-person movement research, enjoy moving in a dance studio with others, chat with the students who frequently drop by my office, or watch live performances in theater seats with others.

As the pandemic rages on, we have also been confronted with a type of racial conflict that has plagued our nation for centuries, but which has been exacerbated by worsening economic conditions and political uncertainty. Some have referred to contemporary racial inequality, the increase in state violence against Black and Brown people, and the racial disparity evinced in Covid-19 death rates and community spread as the *double pandemic*[2] of racial inequity. While Black and Brown people continue to die at higher rates than Whites under the pandemic, they also suffer from a barrage of police assaults, which have left George Floyd, Breonna Taylor, and countless others dead. This inflamed anxiety, fear, and suffering continued alongside an unprecedented attack never before seen in modern U.S. history. On January 6, 2021, a riotous group of Trump supporters attacked the Capitol Building in Washington, D.C., at the behest of the outgoing president. Fearing for their lives, many representatives and staffers hid under desks, while others were forced into secure locations. The violent legions of former President Trump supporters discarded the findings of the mainstream press, the state boards of elections, and the nation's judicial system. Instead, they believed the former president's narrative that the election was stolen from him and were willing to fight the installation of President-elect Biden as president by any means necessary.

As I write this book in the midst of this pandemic and the sociopolitical divides in this country, the influence of implicit biases—those everyday, common occurrences, assumptions, "truths," ways of life, and pervasive beliefs—are either disintegrating or becoming more visible. In the dance world, to speak of holding a dance audition in this historical moment of Covid-19 restrictions no longer means physically traveling to visit the institution. It does not assume auditioning means to dance alongside other auditionees in one location. Instead, it means very different things in various locales across the country from virtual video conference participation to mail-in video footage, to in-person attendance six feet apart while wearing a mask that covers the nose and mouth. To take dance class no longer means I am traveling to a dance studio to move, share, and connect with others in the same room. It instead means I will take a few steps from one area in my home to the computer to participate virtually alongside other boxes of people on a computer screen. Watching a dance performance, in this moment, means watching a screen while comments scroll along the sides, allowing audience members to share their experience. Even the images of normal, everyday life now involve people wearing masks. I can remember before the pandemic, how the oddity of seeing a person in a mask might lead me to wonder why they wore one to begin with. My impulse now is to wonder not only why the person who isn't wearing one is not, but also about their political leanings.

This time of upheaval is the moment in which I am writing this book. I share it as part of the historical context in which I write, a significant influence on how this book came to be what it is, a part of the environment from which it was formed. The Covid-19 pandemic and Black Lives Matter protests of 2020–2021 are part of this book's foundations and influences. During this writing process, with so much loss and suffering, I consider myself fortunate to not only be able to write, but to also be able to interrogate the many assumptions I previously held through my research and this moment in history. There is certainly discomfort for some that comes with the missteps that assumptions produce. However, even in this moment in which we are experiencing a massive and profound disruption of all things normative, there is still deep learning, reflection, and discoveries about myself, about others, and about dance to be had.

This spirit of interpersonal exchange and welcome disruption of cultural norms is also how I ask that you read this book. I intend this book to be a starting point for discussion, a seed from which to ask more questions and learn more about ourselves, our colleagues, and our students. This book is essentially an integration of embodied, textual, and action research on implicit bias and how it manifests in dance education. This term comes from another academic field, the quantitative world of social science. I then examine implicit bias and its effects in our qualitative, embodied, artistic world of dance. The research and workshops I have developed throughout the course of my research investigate implicit bias in dance education in classroom practices, administrative procedures, interpersonal and cultural dynamics, as well as embodied practice. This book offers a new perspective on how to view and reflect upon dance education in hopes that it generates new discoveries, new debates, and new questions. Because this intersection is not yet a central theoretical frame in the field of dance education, I offer it as a way to open possibilities instead of new single, definitive answers. I do not intend this book to be prescriptive in describing exactly what the relationship between implicit bias and dance education is or is not. This book also does not provide formulaic fixes that apply in all dance communities or for all marginalized identities in a way that replication of exercises would be a one-size-fits-all solution to correct the problems that implicit bias presents.

Instead, I introduce this new framework as a way to raise new questions about implicit bias in dance education. I ask, what can now be asked with this new frame that was not a question before? What research methods, new education structures, activities or protocols can be tested in dance classrooms, dance studio businesses, or educational institutions to better understand the role of implicit bias in dance education? What are the experiences and nuanced distinctions about how implicit biases manifest for those that have other identities I have no lived experience of? I hope that this book inspires educators to play, to creatively generate practices, and dialogue about how to be more inclusive, accepting, and open to new perspectives, tastes, and cultural knowledge in the spaces that dance education happens.

Book Chapter Layout

The introduction provides a basic introduction to the social science concepts, structures, and phenomena that define implicit bias and how they manifest in the world of dance education. Chapter 1 explains the power dynamics that undergird the social construction of implicit biases with specific examples of this from dance education. This chapter utilizes the lens of critical theory, which describes the foundations and operation of inequity in the U.S., to better explain why all biases are not equal in society. In Chapters 2 and 3, I focus on particular dynamics of how socialization, systems of power, and aesthetics inform the world of dance and by extension dance education. Chapter 4 provides a variety of examples of implicit biases and their ramifications in the field of dance education. The following chapter, Chapter 5, delves into the mechanisms that exacerbate and those that disrupt the negative effects of implicit biases. In Chapter 6 I describe possible ideas to disrupt inequitable and unwanted effects of implicit bias in classrooms and interactions in dance education that happen outside of the classroom. Lastly, the concluding Chapter 7 returns to a reintegration of the ideas shared in the book by way of specific examples taken from classrooms designed to address both implicit bias while engaging students in research on social justice. It also illuminates the benefits of embodied and reflective processes in uncovering how personal biases manifest in daily dance education environments.

Throughout the book, there are proposed activities located in the breakout sections that offer the reader a moment to engage in an activity that either deepens the exploration of the concept, or offers a moment of reflection on your personal connections to the ideas shared. They are placed at locations throughout the book where the discussions I introduce relate to the physical or reflective engagement. These activities are not only for the reader of this book, but can also be lifted and applied in classroom settings as part of class activities. They can be used to explore the specific topics they relate to in the book—i.e., naming your own biases, developing empathy, or finding new associations and categories for seemingly unrelated objects—or some other creative connection for which you find them useful.

Also throughout the book are somatic check-in moments in which I will ask you to check in with your body by stopping to breathe, journal, or notice any sensations in your body. There may be other places in reading the book that you feel called to engage in this type of somatic check-in. I welcome you to do so as needed. This is an important task in taking in some of the material in the book. As explained later in the book, having a settled body or awareness of your somatic response to something you have read is part of the learning process. It is my hope that this book inspires enduring curiosity, openness, and celebration of the deep and ever unfolding discoveries the work of dance education offers to each one of us as dancers, dance enthusiasts, members of the field of dance, and citizens of the world.

Introduction
Biases and Behavior

I want to begin with a confession. I have biases. My favorite color is blue, and I prefer a chocolate-vanilla swirl in my soft-serve ice cream. I used to prefer straight, long, flowy hair growing up, but now I much prefer my own natural kinks and curls; hair that grows up, not down. In my daily attire, I have a bias for the loose-fitting, flowy pants I have spent so many years in the dance studio wearing. Tight jeans, power suits, or formal wear feel much too restrictive for what I would like to do with my moving body throughout the day. I prefer pants over dresses and avoid make-up mostly as a revolt from the beauty pageants my mother raised me in starting at the age of two.

My dance biases are a strong love of postmodern dance. This love for postmodern dance is for its penchant for disrupting and questioning norms and signals of status quo, its affinity for discovering new possibilities that dare the creator, dancer, and audience to rethink everything they know. I also have a strong inclination for dance ethnography and the myriad dances of the African diaspora and East Indian diaspora. In terms of educational pedagogy, I am biased towards the dialogic and civic orientation of Maxine Greene's inspiring and philosophical work in aesthetic education. I am biased toward engendering in students' imagination a creative sense of their own personal life experiences and how advocating for their voice and for the voice of others is part of civic, democratizing citizenship. In my own gender identity associations, I prefer the gender pronouns of she, her, and they.

In the embodied anti-racism workshops I facilitate, this sharing exercise is often how I begin the discussion about biases in dance education. Some of these biases, i.e., my love of the color blue, may seem inconsequential. Others, like my preference for postmodern dance, may feel more like defining significant factors that help you to understand a bit about what is to come and who I am as the author of this book. I share these partly for you to have a sense of my positionality as author of this book. Sharing positionality statements[1] facilitates a more equitable and inclusive environment for critical discussion and understanding. Another reason I share some of my biases is to exhibit more of a whole person, to evoke personal connection between you and me. A third reason I share these biases is to demonstrate that not only do I have them, but also everyone has biases. Also, sharing some of my biases serves as a model for taking ownership of them, to clear the deception that I can ever really be completely impartial. Biases affect how humans see themselves and the world around them. It is part of what connects people who have similar biases, affinities, or aversions. In some cases, it divides people who share different sensibilities. In addition, it simply aids in people having a clearer understanding of the perspectives of others and how those perspectives stem from their lived experiences.

Naming your biases can also be a regular practice to develop a capacity for owning them and illuminating those biases for others. In the workshops I conduct, I then expand into a bias-related identity exploration activity to be added to the list of other identity exploration activity ideas that come later in this book. Participants of the sessions I facilitate and the classes I teach are asked to share some of their biases with each other in smaller groups. They are asked to reflect and share which preferences or aversions feel significant and which do not. This bias sharing activity serves as an icebreaker and trust exercise for developing participant connection and deeper understanding of each other. Not only does it encourage getting to know each other, but it is also a way to unearth reflective realizations about how an individual's biases they are aware of inform their daily lives in meaningful ways.

A valuable place to start to examine the role that biases play in everyday life would be to keep a running list of the conscious biases you hold over an extended period of time. Then reflect and assign whether you feel each bias is one of personal significance in how you navigate the world or whether you feel it inconsequential. After you have kept this running list for some time, look back over some of the earlier biases you contributed to the list. Have they changed or morphed over time? Are there some that have changed in significance over time? The abbreviated version of this exercise I facilitate in workshops addresses **explicit biases**. These *explicit biases* are likes, dislikes, and associations that I can articulate and that I know consciously. There are also **implicit biases**. An *implicit bias* is a like, dislike, or association that a person does not consciously know they have and cannot articulate. Both of these types of biases affect how people think about the world they live in, who they are in that environment, and how they decide to navigate the world. In short, biases affect how we perceive the world and ourselves in the world.

ACTIVITY BOX #1: Naming Your Biases

What are some of your biases you are aware of? List out as many as you can. You may find it helpful to think in terms of categories in order to make your list as robust as possible. For example, what are some of your food biases or fashion biases, dance biases, or daily routine or house organization biases? What are the biases that feel rather unimportant or insignificant in terms of how they affect your daily life? What are the biases that feel significant either to how you think of yourself as a person, educator, or dancer? What are the biases that feel significant to your perspective as a dancer?

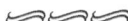

Furthermore, what humans perceive isn't solely what the senses gather, but also what meaning the brain-body[2] makes of this sensory information. This is not new information for those who are brain game enthusiasts, who have seen the paintings where other images pop out of them if you stare long enough or watch the television series *Brain Games*.[3] The implication of these glitches[4] in human brains is often presented as a functional adjustment that better supports some evolutionary challenge the mind must address for the success of the species. So much of how brains function and adapt to the environment is either unknown in the areas of expert research or unnoticed by individuals as the brain does its work.[5] The brain often operates so well that we do not notice many of the aspects of how it is functioning. Yet many can certainly concede to the brain's function having profound effects on how people navigate the world. Much of how the brain sorts and organizes the massive amounts of information it takes in is through categorization.

The Meaning-Making Process

Carol-Lynne Moore and Kaoru Yamamoto articulate the process of observation, categorization, and meaning-making in *Beyond Words: Movement Observation and Analysis*.[6] The authors take the reader on a journey along what the authors call the "Ladder of Abstraction."[7] In this metaphorical ladder model, the human brain-body experiences the world, then groups similar experiences into more generalized categories that become more and more abstract conceptually. The brain-body processes experiences of the world by collecting massive amounts of sensory information, seeking out patterns and ways to categorize the information, and making meaning to understand and even predict aspects of what is happening in the environment. Many of these systems of organization are intimately linked to our biases and categories provided by our social environment.

A rather humorous and articulate way to explain biases comes from the world of comedy. During the time I was researching for this book I took what I thought was a break to watch Daniel Sloss' 2020 HBO comedy special, *Daniel Sloss: X*.[8] The research, however, ended up following me into this experience. Part of the comedy special included a segment where Sloss speaks about a character named Nigel living inside his brain. Sloss explained how this character is the name given to the cataloger or archivist in his mind that maintains the memories of old and often outdated beliefs Sloss has not examined since they were formed. Because the beliefs have not been examined in some time, Sloss relayed how he was now rather embarrassed to still carry around some of the beliefs.

Aside from the segment's comedic entertainment, I found this to be a rather great metaphor for what happens inside the brain with **implicit memories**. *Implicit memory*[9] is when recollections of past experiences influence later performance with no recognition of the past experience and its effect on that later performance.[10] Essentially, the brain-body is recollecting without consciously realizing it is recollecting or even what memory or memories it is remembering. The idea of there being an archival attendant that can pull out the beliefs developed in the course of a person's life, dust them off to determine what opinion a person might have seemed to resonate, as effective comedy skits often do, with something real and true in daily life. Sloss continued with this metaphor to explain the moment of cringeful reflex that ensues when he realizes the belief that Nigel points out is still archived and is embarrassingly outdated to how Sloss thinks about the world in the present. This aspect of the unconscious mind illustrates in simple and comedic terms how implicit memories and beliefs still exist in the mind with little awareness of their existence until a moment arises to call that attitude into active engagement or application in a situation. Further resonance takes place in Sloss' account of a disconnect between present-day consciousness and the unconscious mind. The present-day consciousness can be rather appalled by these antiquated beliefs still lingering in the unconscious mind.

Take, for example, our explicit biases. Some are personal preferences that are based on the individual's personal passions, attractions, and aversions that don't align with anyone else that they know. For instance, there is a rather common discussion I experience in dance classes about bare feet. A student may have an aversion to touching feet or removing their socks in a dance class. I have had these conversations negotiating with students about their discomfort stemming from this explicit bias against exposed bare feet from elementary through high school. Other preferences and aversions fit very squarely within the group or groups a person identifies with. For example, people who have an affinity for rebellious representations in art or life may like rock and roll or some other form of music that seems to be representative of a certain sensibility of rebelliousness. Also, what is culturally uncommon such as an aversion to touching feet in one culture, may be a common, normative aversion in another culture. For example, a culture like some contexts I encountered during my time in Rajasthan, India, may have an established norm that touching people's feet is offensive, unclean, or taboo. In another cultural context it may be deemed a sign of respect for elders in the culture. Biases are something every person has, as it is a mechanism in which the brain makes sense of the world.

The Negative Effects of Bias

What becomes problematic at the very least and damaging at most is when individuals are not aware of how their biases are affecting how they navigate the world. Think of a bias as a personal perspective based on the lived experiences of one individual. For example, I might personally find long fingernails a nuisance because I am unable to manipulate items in my hand the same way when I have long nails as I do when I do not have long nails. Now think of that bias as a consistent and universal truth or fact. Shifting the nail example into a universal truth might then mean that long nails are a poor choice for everyone because it means the person is unproductive and ineffective at navigating daily tasks because the long nails interfere for everyone who has them. This extends into hiring practices, where applicants with long nails are not hired based on the logic established when the individual perspective shifted into applying to other people. This misrepresentation of a bias as factual or indisputable truth is one negative effect. It is problematic because it is a misapplication of a bias where a bias has been applied to a situation as a rule or truth. From the world of dance, you can think about biases such as that music must be part of a dance performance, or that a student in higher education who is learning to make dances benefits from not using music to create the dance, or that because ballet is a foundational technique for the dance forms of your experience, that it is a form that is foundational for all dance forms.

Another negative effect is the expectation that others should have this same perspective in order to be accepted, legitimate, or appropriate representations of the community. Biases influence what one holds to be true, right or wrong, valuable or worthless, or how a person thinks of themselves or others. When a person with privileges or dominant social status is given free reign, even the most harmless of biases can take root not as a simple preference, but as some sort of collective truth or rule that others must comply with. This operation of bias within social power structures can become a dangerous misrepresentation or a power-laden concept, especially in dance studios and classrooms.

Un-Biased: The God-Trick

So much power and privilege has gone to systems and fields of study that purport to be neutral, objective, and unbiased. The field of social science has done significant research in determining the role implicit bias has in previously purported unbiased systems.[11] These fields and systems have benefited from a societal privilege and bestowing of power to systems that assert claims of objectivity and impartiality. The list of fields spans from law to journalism and publication houses, to the sciences, technology, engineering, and math (STEM), to medicine, sports referees, and to the most visibly deadly in the current historical moment, law enforcement.

When claims of impartiality come from members of a socially dominant segment of society and thus are accepted to have veracity, there is a perception of *Truth*, of **testimonial bias** that comes with that assertion.[12] *Testimonial bias* is a type of implicit bias for who a person believes or finds reputable and who they do not. These determinations of who is worthy of trust are not as readily based on factual discernment as previously thought, and instead are based on what systems of knowledge a person trusts. For example, a person may trust information from family members more than academic scholars, their studio instructor more than the judges from the television show *So You Think You Can Dance*. In society, systems that claim impartiality are often imbued with more power or veracity of perspective than say, dance artists. The very notion of objectivity or impartiality in society functions as a signal of having more prominent value assigned to their findings. Of course, some of this empirical and objective examination and research is valuable and even useful in detecting when biases are influencing those systems. But social sciences have revealed these systems are not quite as unbiased as they purport to be.

For example, in the U.S. justice system, Justin Levinson's[13] research on misremembering of testimony during trial jury deliberation bears out racial bias as jurors attempt to recollect the objective evidence of cases. He explains how racial biases affect what jurors remember and how it results in either remembering inaccurately or not remembering some aspects at all. For example, a juror may remember a Black person being the aggressor in a testimonial account when the court record, once reviewed, documented the testimony indicating the Black person was the victim, not the aggressor. Because of the socialization that Black people are prone to violence, a juror may have what Levinson calls a *misremembrance* of the account given in the trial during deliberations. Cheryl Harris eloquently writes about how the operation of *White* as a racial category is so critical to the privilege of being believed and of innocence that she lays out the overwhelming evidence in the legal system of Whiteness functioning as an unspoken, implicit property right similar to other legal rights within the law.[14]

So, in what way are these systems unbiased? As an example of what demographic data can illuminate, consider that the U.S. population in 2019, according to the U.S. Census, puts those who identify as Black in the national population at 13.4 percent and those who identify as White in the U.S. population at 76.3 percent.[15] Below are demographic statistics in each of the above-mentioned fields.[16]

Lawyers: 5.9 percent Black; 86.6 percent White
Judges and other judicial occupations[17]: 13.4 percent Black; 81.5 percent White
Reporters, correspondents, and analysts: 6.9 percent Black; 82.4 percent White
Publishing industry: 5 percent Black; 75 percent White[18]
Engineering and Architecture occupations: 6.8 percent Black; 77.5 percent White
Social, physical, and life sciences: 6.3 percent Black; 76.9 percent White
Mathematics and computer occupations: 8.7 percent Black; 65.7 percent White
Medical doctors: 3.42 percent Black; 79.5[19]
Athletes, umpires, coaches, and related occupations: 9.3 percent Black; 81.1 percent White
Education, library, and training occupations: 10.2 percent Black; 81.7 percent White
Police officers[20]: 12.8 percent Black; 65.5 percent White
Choreographers and dancers: 6.73 percent Black; 67 percent White[21]

If these are the statistics of employment in these fields that purport some attention to objectivity and impartiality, it is important to consider the possibility of, and in some cases proven, biases (in this case racial bias) that go unnamed, unacknowledged, or unexamined. The most conservative of conclusions from this data shows there is evidence of inequitable representation at the very least. Yet, these institutions of culture and society purport to be objective and unbiased in aspects of decision-making, analysis, and knowledge-creation. If we are to include consideration and deliberation of who is accepted into these fields, the representation statistics of these fields exhibit a different narrative. This alternate narrative provides evidence of historical exclusion of people who self-identify as Black in these fields and points to evidence of a possible bias in the deliberations for these positions in these fields. The demographic breakdown of the field of dance and dance education is further detailed in the data collected from the National Association of Schools of Dance (NASD).

As an example of how dance programs and organizations can track data, I have sourced the NASD 2018–2019 Higher Education Arts Data Services (HEADS) with regards to racial demographics in undergraduate student, graduate student, and faculty/instructor data reported during the 2018–2019 academic year.[22] First, a significant factor is how many schools reported. In order to have the most accurate information available, all possible data must be collected. In this report, the highest percentage of NASD schools that reported data was 74 percent of the institutions accredited by NASD. While this is a large majority of the schools who reported and statistically substantial and adequate for data collection, it would be a fuller, more accurate representation of the affiliated organizations with 100 percent of schools reporting. Also, NASD-accredited programs are by no means a representation of the entire field of dance in the U.S. when considering public primary and secondary school programs, dance companies with teaching artist programs, independent small business dance studios, and various dance organizations and groups that are organized around an ethnic or national identity outside of the U.S. dominant culture. Finally, it would be significant to determine how the racial data was collected. Are participants self-identifying, or are administrators determining via visual and/or secondary resources to assign race?

The next aspect of the data that was noticeable is 28.6 percent of Visiting Faculty were noted to be Black or African American of all Visiting Faculty hired at the institutions, whereas 11.7 percent of full Professors were reported to be Black or African American. Inversely, 52.4 percent of Visiting Faculty were identified as White, whereas 75.8 percent of full Professors were reported to be White. When you compare these statistics to the national average pulled from the U.S. Census statistics, there is a disproportionate correlation. The U.S. Census estimates the 2019 national percentages of self-identified Black or African American people at 13.4 percent and national percentages of self-identified White people at 76.3 percent. It is noticeable that those hired in the temporary faculty position of Visiting Faculty tend to be above the national average of Black faculty and significantly below the national average of White people hired in Visiting Faculty positions. For the Professor positions, the number of reported White faculty holds relatively close to the national percentage of White people in the U.S. The number of reported Black faculty in the position of Professor dips below the national percentage of Black people in the U.S. providing evidence of the marginalized status of Black dancers in tenure-track positions.[23]

ACTIVITY BOX #2: Imagining Futures

What would diversity, equity, and inclusion look like in dance programs from your perspective? Be as detailed as possible. In the first pass at this exploration, do not consider the blocks or reasons this has not or cannot be implemented. Simply describe what a diverse, equitable, and inclusive dance program looks like for you. After this first pass, you may then begin to look at the deterrents, histories and reasons for the "why nots."

In seeking to understand the context of this dataset, it is important to further examine the factors that are in play. As with the data gleaned from the quantitative studies of social psychologists, the data can only illuminate a very specific set of information addressing a very specific set of questions. It is up to those of us in the qualitative fields to make sense of these elements in the lived experiences of the field, students, and ourselves as educators. For example, this set of data aligns with the assertion that Black people are not as often granted full ownership status in a metaphorical land ownership model of the field of dance education. Rather, White supremacist structures establish that Whiteness is the standard that receives ownership status with the rights that ownership imbues, while Black dancers and dance educators are relegated to renter status, to be moved around the field at the will of the standards, goals, and agendas set by permanent full-time institution members and systemic structures of Whiteness.[24]

In this climate in the field of dance, the concept of bias, as it relates to this phenomenon of ownership in the field and a sense of belonging, has come up in a number of discussions. Chyrstyn Mariah Fentroy[25] describes her lived experiences as a Black ballerina with biases that people she has encountered unknowingly carry and apply to her and other dancers of color. In a *Dance Magazine* Op-ed article[26] Theresa Ruth Howard establishes a case for addressing the negative effects of bias in dance criticism. Courtney Celeste Spears reveals ways for students to confront the negative effects of bias in studio dance settings in a 2020 *Dance Spirit* article.[27] In 2020 Riis Williams published an article about the work the Pacific Northwest Ballet has been doing to combat bias in representation of its dancers and what work there is still to do.[28] These are only a fraction of the discussions around bias in dance in popular publications. As these examples demonstrate, conversations of belonging and bias in dance extend beyond the exclusive environments of the myriad publications in academic journals that cost money to access that educational institutions provide.

Take, for example, the U.S. dance education field's well-established bias for ballet and modern dance. Consider what the field of dance education might look like if this bias was contextualized as only a preference of a number of members of the community instead of being applied as "the foundation of all dance."[29] From this stance, it serves as the mechanism for determining whether students are successful or talented dancers. What might the training structure of other dance forms look like if the methods and structures of ballet and modern dance were not applied to the pedagogies of other forms? How might curriculum, assessment, or student selection change if the assessment was based on evaluative systems that did not orient toward examining the execution of specifically named vocabularies and instead was based on criteria aligned with other dance forms? What might the economic structures of program funding look like if dance forms other than ballet and modern dance were funded at the same numbers throughout the course of the field's growth by funders who had a bias for dance forms beyond ballet and modern? How might financial access for students be affected by different requirements as it relates to dance studio dress based on dance forms that think differently than ballet and modern dance about what clothing is needed for dance class?

This question extended from an experience I had listening to social science researcher Dr. Mahzarin Banaji present at the National Association of Independent Schools' People of Color Conference in 2015. Listening to her share her lived experiences opened up an entirely new perspective on those evolutionarily useful glitches in human brains that result in implicit biases negatively affecting human behavior. I had already read the book she co-authored, *Blindspot: Hidden Biases of Good People*, a book I still highly recommend. It was through the in-person interaction, the dynamic activities, and personal stories I will detail further later in the book that the implications of her work became so very clear. Succinctly put, there are mechanisms in the human brain that cause us to categorize information gleaned from human interactions based on data collected from our previous experiences without any awareness this processing is happening. These categorizations determine decisions, social judgments, understandings, concepts of self, and actions taken daily.

The results of these cognitive organizational frameworks are referred to as *implicit attitudes* or *implicit bias*. It takes a counterproductive, harmful turn when the data collected from previous experiences may have been created based on a dataset oriented toward an already established misconception or applied to an inappropriate context. In other words, a false truth about some groups of people, a poignant experience, or event being applied to future events that are unrelated. These flawed datasets result in experiences and details being thrown out of the brain's consciousness if the details do not align with the narrative and interpretations already existent in the brain. This is the process of misremembering mentioned above in Levinson's work.

The human brain is so fast and so efficient that this happens often without the perceiver even realizing this process is taking place. It happens before the conscious brain that controls executive functioning has time to engage with the data coming into the brain. We move through life with certainty that our history and our collected datasets are accurate and applicable for the foreseeable future. This is the frame of socialization. The way any human is taught and raised to view the world is the guiding organization for creating meaning and understanding these data sets in childhood. Not until a person develops opposing experiences or skills to critically question those foundational beliefs does the frame of perception tend to change. Even then, without becoming aware of these implicit biases or making intentional adjustments in daily practice, these biases can continue to shape what a person believes to be a logical and objective decision, perception, or behavior. This is why people with higher levels of education score no differently in terms of having bias, but rather have a lower instance of endorsing having bias.[30]

As a dancer and educator, I found this idea intriguing. When I think of the ephemeral, ever-disappearing moments of watching and performing dance, the idea of brain glitches in what the brain processes and integrates into the body frightens me. The level of potential misinformation and misprocessing, with no way to undo the moment that just took place or even realize it happened, is rife with capacity for falsehood. This all occurs while the brain assures the perceiver that it has effectively done its job. Based on the findings of implicit bias research, serious consideration must be taken that in dance studios there are brains of teachers, adjudicators, colleagues miscategorizing or discarding aspects of movement or behavior to the detriment of a student, candidate, or colleague. How are biases feeding into our understanding of a dancer, a student, an educator, a leader? What is happening in classrooms in the moments of observation and assessment? How are we to track the effects of bias in classroom discussion for students or colleagues for which there are little to no ways to provide evidence and, thus, illuminate patterns of teacher biases in student behavior, contributions, or academic performance in that classroom setting?

Because of the power of vision, a predominant human sense, visually taking in information and assessing it is one of the most prevalent ways that biases affect attitudes toward people, decisions made, and behaviors particularly in dance, a field so oriented toward visual experiences of the body.[31] While at times, there is a confluence of sensory experiences that provides data for cognitive processes to make sense of our experience, the visual markers of what are seen are the quickest and most potent way that biases are both formed and reinforced. For this reason, in this book I will spend more time attending to those identity markers that are more visually apparent. As a researcher of how racism manifests in dance education, more attention and more application of how implicit bias affects the dance studios and classrooms will focus on race. As the book unveils the effects of implicit bias and how it manifests, it will become more and more apparent that the construct of race is one of the many considerations that contribute to implicit biases. Because these categories are myriad and interconnected, I will focus on visual identifiers, as they most often contribute to how students are assessed in the classrooms and studios of dance education.

As with any new frame of organization, exploration, or line of inquiry, when there is potential for great failure, there is also potential for great learning and discovery. How can dance educators track these implicit biases, catch these glitches in teaching and professional interactions? In what ways can an understanding of these implicit biases help students, educators, and administrators engage in dialogue that is generative and illuminating about unspoken assumptions operating in dance programs, businesses, and organizations? This book is about exploring both sides of this coin in the context of dance education, in studios, classrooms, and administrative spaces of dance learning. It includes not only explanations of how implicit biases affect dance education settings, but also offers strategies for upending the negative effects of both implicit and explicit biases in community. The purpose of this exploration is to generate future ideas and applications in the field of dance on how to reprogram the brain-body to be more equitable and inclusive in its perceptions and collection of datasets to create more equitable and inclusive results in dance education programs and communities.

Working Terminology

Current research in social psychology has provided us with new points to consider in how this prejudicial process works in the hard-wiring of the brain. **Implicit social cognition** is the area of study where the concept of implicit bias was coined with over 20 years of research dedicated to this area.[32] *Implicit social cognition* refers to the unconscious, automatic, or implicit processes that underlie judgments and social behavior. It is a broad area of study that affects self-esteem, concepts of self, social judgment, social cognitive development, goal pursuit, romantic relationships, decision making, prejudice, stereotyping, and social justice. For this reason, the effects of this area of study have been applied in a number of sectors including the criminal justice system, businesses in their hiring and worker evaluation practices, commercial marketing and sales, and of course the education sector to name a few.

There are two areas of implicit social cognition I will focus on in this book. One is implicit memory, the other, implicit attitudes. In philosophy, implicit memories are connected with the concept of aesthetics as "what is perceptible" or "the sensible" meaning taken in or experienced by the senses.[33] In dance, an example of this might be a dance educator posting images of ballerinas en pointe in her studio over and over that are experienced in passing by everyone who enters the space. This could be broaches, posters, ceramic interior decorations, clothing of or with ballerinas, etc., that are taken in without bringing the student's attention to having this reference in eye view. Then ask students, for whom this is their most prominent experience of dance, to name a form of dance or even their favorite form of dance. Unless the student has a strong exposure or preference for a different form, or a strong experiential disrupter exposing the student to a different dance form, the student will most likely name ballet due to the ***priming*** of exposure to ballet. *Priming* in the field of psychology is exposing a person or persons to a stimulus that affects human behavior but without conscious awareness by the person affected that the stimulus has affected their behavior.[34] Researchers are able to detect changes in behavior that occur once a person is primed even though those they are researching are unaware of the change.

One of the changes that a person is unaware of is their implicit attitudes. Implicit attitudes refer to the evaluative associations or characterizations a person holds toward a person or group of people based on past experiences that inform or affect future behavior. This occurs when people are either unaware of the association or the source of that association. These past experiences can be individual experiences or culturally collective messaging or social cues. An implicit attitude often relates to socially constructed categories taken for granted in society. Examples of these associations include categories of ability, class, gender, race, religion, sexuality, or weight. An example of this might be the attitude or preference that male-identifying and female-identifying ballroom dancers pair together because of social cues that privilege heterosexual pairings as affectional preferences.

An area of attention for this book in studies of implicit attitudes is **bias**. Defining features of *biases* addressed in this book were gleaned from critical theory and defined more specifically as *preferences or inclinations developed from preconceived opinions*.[35] Some of these preferences are reflective, conscious, and explicit. These explicit biases are based on aspects of personal experience one can explicitly articulate. Many dancers, for example, have a bias for movement. In other words, they find movement a pleasurable experience. To have an explicit bias for dance would mean being able to articulate your love for dance. For example, maybe you are from a family of dancers, or you saw a performance that inspired your love and passion for dance. In this way, you are able to link your past experiences or memories to your present love for dance.

Implicit bias is another form of bias that is automatic and stems from cultural norms, assumptions, and other past experiences that are linked to implicit memories. As a result, the person is unaware of the experiences and memories from which the biases stem. Even once the holder of the bias becomes aware of the bias, the person may still be unable to determine why they hold that particular bias or even be unable to track its effects, the implicit memories, or their personal preferences, aversions, decisions, and behaviors.

Evolutionarily speaking, this is useful to the brain's ability to process, which allows for quick reactions based on collective assessments of past experiences without taking large amounts of time in the moment to discern what actions to take or to avoid taking. It is certainly instrumental in how the human brain-body learns and adapts. Once a habit of mind is embedded, there is a quicker response time without the brain-body having to go through the steps it had to in earlier stages of learning. Reading these words on the page, for example, are happening at a quicker pace than early attempts to read, because the brain-body has developed quicker pathways to enact the activity without returning to each step of the complexities of what it takes to read.

This is also how **culture** is formed, through these habitual messages, practices, and beliefs. Psychotherapist and somatic abolitionist educator Resmaa Menakem defines *culture* as

> how our bodies retain and reenact history—through the foods we eat (or refuse to eat); the stories we tell; the things that hold meaning for us; the images that move us; what we are able (and unable) to sense or feel or process; the way we see the world; and a thousand other aspects of life.[36]

Significant to the way in which I will be discussing culture as it relates to the work of upending the negative effects of bias is what he goes on to articulate about culture in the body. Menakem states, "Because culture lives in our bodies, it usually trumps all things cognitive—ideas, philosophies, convictions, principles, and laws."[37] The body is where culture lives, is shared with others, and is habituated and passed on from generation to generation. This is how it supersedes cognitive activity. When we teach dance, we are introducing students to particular cultural dispositions and sensibilities through the moving body.

Watching students in the learning process discover some of those integral aspects of learning a complex concept is one of my favorite moments as a teacher. It helps me appreciate and not take for granted the aspects I now know but have forgotten that I once had to learn in small, incremental steps. These embedded, habitual sensibilities happen in discerning human interactions based on previous messaging and experiences as well. However, when the messages and experiences received are flawed, inaccurate, or misrepresent reality, this process becomes profoundly problematic at best and dangerous at worst.

An old and pervasive example of a cultural norm that has a well-established record of implicit messages and memories that are injected into the subconscious minds of those living in the U.S. is the example of racial categories. In the U.S. we are inundated with messages that signal White bodies (visually marked by having white or melanin-lacking skin) are the standard, higher caste, dominant group in the socialization model of the U.S. Black bodies (visually marked by having black or brown melanin-rich skin) are at the bottom of that hierarchy as the substandard, lowest caste, stigmatized, or marginalized group distinctly separate from and opposite of the standard of White skin.[38] Those that are categorized as Asian, Pacific Islander, Native American, or other socially constructed regional, ethnic, and religious identities such as Jewish, Middle Eastern, Latinx, Arab, Hispanic, etc., also often are ascribed a stigmatized status in similar, yet complex and shifting ways in relation to White bodies as the standard. Resmaa Menakem refers to this as "White-body supremacy," describing it as "the equivalent of a toxic chemical we ingest on a daily basis. Eventually, it changes our brains and the chemistry of our bodies."[39]

What is so complex about this is how perception shapes reality. While we may understand consciously that race is a social construct that is not real or accurate, we live in a world that biases, behaviors, and institutions have created in which the construct operates as reality and certainly feels real for so many on the stigmatizing end of these social constructs. Take, for example, the earlier demographic information shared on percentages of those who identify as White and Black in various careers. Tracking the quantitative data of how individuals identify racially in those fields may feel like it exhibits some scientific truth about race. In reality, what it indicates is a social phenomenon, the results unveiling how the assumptions, perceptions, and stereotypes held in a pervasive way in this country affect career and class status based on racial categories. It quantitatively signals not any truth about race as some sort of biological human characteristic, but rather signals a social phenomenon of what we believe about racial distinctions in this country. In this way, those stigmatized by discrimination and marginalization based on their race feel the lived reality of this invented social construct. Those privileged by the construct may be able to evade facing the inaccuracies, inequities, and social detriment of race as a construct, as the social structure is designed to make such inequity invisible and comfortable to evade.

These biases can take a variety of forms in the field of dance education and can vary depending on genre, professional context of the dance class, or locale. For example, an individual may find taller dancers more pleasant to watch, because of exposure to concert dance forms that either prefer or require dancers to be a certain height. Another could be finding classical, elongated movement of ballet unpleasant because the viewer grew up watching percussive dance forms such as tap. Yet another might be encouraging Asian-identifying dancers to pursue dance forms that stem from Asian cultures, because the teacher makes the assumption that such dancers prefer forms that correlate with their racial identity.

Some implicit biases contradict the reflective, conscious biases that exist in the body-mind of one single individual. When faced with a moment where an implicit bias conflicts with an explicit bias the uncomfortable sensation or feeling of **cognitive dissonance** can take place.[40] *Cognitive dissonance* is the disquieting sensation that occurs when a person becomes aware that an unconscious bias is operating that conflicts with the conscious beliefs the person has. Becoming aware of implicit biases, Banaji and Greenwald state, "causes distress, even sadness, because it undermines the image we have of ourselves as largely fair-minded and egalitarian."[41]

In response to this melancholy or discomfort, the brain often resolves this disconnect by interpreting experiences in ways that align with existing beliefs. This phenomenon is called **confirmation bias**.[42] *Confirmation bias* is a systematic processing in our brains that deems those things that do not fit into our belief systems to be anomalies, outliers, or faulty information. Take, for example, an implicit bias that short dancers are less articulate dancers alongside an explicit belief that height does not matter in determining whether a dancer is an articulate mover. The mind begins to interpret what it experiences as evidence that supports the implicit belief that the short dancer is not articulate. This way, the mind can continue to hold on to an explicit belief that height does not determine the articulation of a dancer's body while also providing "evidence" that, in this particular case, the "data proves" this dancer is not articulate.

Confirmation bias is a way to maintain the belief system that is in place. Levinson's concept of misremembrances discussed earlier is another example of this tendency of the brain to either discard or alter information taken in that does not align with implicit biases. The cognitive operation is metaphorically similar to the quantitative world's graphing of a set of data points, then choosing the threshold at which outliers are excluded from consideration of the main data set. Key to these new discoveries is the fact that individuals are completely unaware that their brain-bodies, in effect, disappear information that does not fit neatly into their belief systems. Furthermore, data shows that those who have a higher level of education statistically are less willing to concede to the fact that they exhibit implicit bias and thus can be more susceptible to confirmation bias.[43] This refusal precipitates a stagnation in disrupting the biases in operation, and by extension maintains the biases the observer refuses to acknowledge.

Recently I was a part of an extensive search process for incoming dancers to an educational organization. The live components of the interview process consisted of a studio movement component, a group discussion with members of the organization and applicants for this position, and an interview with the search team which I was a part of. I noticed in the interview portion of this search that the notes I had taken prior to the interview seemed to be further substantiated in my analysis of candidate responses in the interview. As the interview was the final portion of this search process, I could not help but question whether the conclusions I came to in the interview were simply how my brain-body organized and categorized the answers provided in such ways that they supported my previous findings. I had a moment of critical reflection, questioning the effectiveness of the interviews if the results were a potential site of confirmation bias wherein my brain sorted how I experienced the answers in a way that aligned with the assessments I already held about the candidates.

This process of activating an implicit bias happens so quickly, as a person observes a dancer moving, that it may not make it to the executive higher levels of cognitive processing where conscious deliberation is made. Isabelle Wilkerson, for example, explains how quickly the implicit negative racial bias some White people have toward Black people functions.[44] Wilkerson states, "Among whites, the sight of a Black person, even in faded yearbook photographs, can trigger the amygdala of the brain to perceive threat and arm itself for vigilance within 30 milliseconds of exposure, the blink of an eye, researchers have found."[45] Consider the way in which dance is taken in, its ephemerality, and the complexities of abstract physical gestures and markers of movement that combine in varying contexts, performances, and bodies to create what the observer sees. The experience of observing, making meaning, and assessing or evaluating movement is a site rich in possibilities to rouse the influence of implicit bias. With so much happening so fast in ways that one often can never replicate exactly that same way again, dance is rife with opportunities for implicit bias to manifest itself.

So where does this acknowledgment of an implicit bias leave a person in terms of discriminatory behavior? Does having a bias automatically make a person a bigot? Not necessarily. But it does make a person more susceptible to reverting to implicit bias-based determinations whenever the person is distracted, fatigued, or lacks ample information to make a more informed decision.[46] As dance educators, the "to do list" to consider in the day and life of teaching—keeping track of time; assessing student performance in class; effectively communicating to the group and individuals in class; holding space for students in crisis; encouraging students who are more apprehensive; classroom management; making connections to previous or future content; tracking student social interactions in class; etc.—is a formidable list to tackle. There are days that feel like successes when dance teachers feel the joy of making connections and celebrating having each student feel seen and acknowledged for who they are. Of course, there are other days when dance teachers know missteps were made in which harm or ill-intended effects took place from momentary choices or language used in curricular instruction. What is key is accepting that at no time will the teaching process ever be perfect all the time. Rather, the process always leans toward improving the quality of dance education and cultivates a sense of belonging among students in the classroom. In order to be better informed about how these seemingly small or inconsequential brain glitches have major effects in the microcosm of the dance studios and dance classrooms, it is key to understand their role in the larger environment of the U.S.

Take, for example, the commitment of dance educators who advocate for marginalized or underrepresented members of the community that also happen to not meet the explicitly stated qualifications. These advocates are often perceived, by themselves and others, to be progressive, forward-thinking, and compassionate dance educators committed to disrupting racism by advocating for underrepresented faculty, guest artists, or students in educational programs. I have observed White disruptors of power systems fiercely advocate for students of color to be accepted into roles for which they do not meet the explicit expectations of selection. These impassioned change-makers have not only advocated for these students, but often provided the additional support for the student or colleague's academic or professional performance when the resulting difficulties evidenced in application materials presented themselves in the academic or professional performance of the candidate.

While this may initially appear to be an anti-racist practice, I propose a different analysis that actually reinforces implicit racial bias tropes. The assumption that the charge to ensure there are more students of color involves accepting students who have not met the explicit benchmarks of the application process involves a bias that students of color perform at lower rates that justify accepting students who do not meet the benchmarks explicitly established by the institution or the program. It also engenders the long-established White savior narrative wherein White people, instead of fighting for equitable treatment and resources prior to student applications, rather establish themselves as the savior figure with an inequitable power dynamic amongst those candidates of color who have been afforded *a favor* to be included. While well-intended, this approach still upholds racist assumptions that people of color are less qualified or capable than White candidates, and that they will need help rather than equitable treatment and access. This is an example of the complex and insidious nature of how fluid, contextual, and entrenched the influence of implicit biases can be on perceptions and behaviors. In order to track these nuances in a multitude of complex and highly context-dependent circumstances, one seeking to deter or disrupt the negative effects of implicit bias must understand the structure of the implicit messages and memories that create the pattern of thought lodged in the subconscious body-mind and how their sense of self-identity relates to those priming messages and sociocultural structures.

Visible Markers and Ascribed Identities

Locations of identity are socially composed and then assigned. This may seem simple and simply-defined. However, because identities imposed by others are constructed over-simplifications, there are always outliers that do belong to the group but for which the categories do not quite seem to fit by the usual markers of the identity. These classifications relayed in the verbal, behavioral, and visual messages received living in the U.S. are used to divide and classify groups of people whether people identify themselves within the category or not. They often ascribe value or privilege along the way, while at the same time may also form social bonds of connection and common experience between those of a social classification.

Take, for example, racial categories. While the brain may register and assign these categories based on visual markers related to the majority of people who identify as one race or another (usually by skin color, hair, and/or facial features), there are people who may identify as a racial category that do not visually present to others as that category. If the racial category of Black is attributed to those with brown skin color and curly hair, there may be people living with hypo-pigmentation conditions such as albinism or people of mixed heritage who identify as Black but who visually do not present as Black-bodied people. In this way, their visual markers of race result in privileges or stigmas they receive from the outside world even if they identify differently than how others see them. Non-disabled bodies are another location of identity that may assume some visible, physical, or behavioral attribute. The classification associated with cognitive abilities often goes unidentified and uncategorized. There are people whose gender expression is not aligned with the heteronormative binary of masculine or feminine making categorization complex in the dominant binary structure of gender or people whose sexuality preference does not present in stereotypical behaviors and bend the heteronormative assumptions of feminine or masculine behavior. These are examples of how visual markers are insufficient to signal identities.

To further the quandary of social categorization and implicit bias, there is the shift that can happen when the disconnect between assumptions based on visual representation of a person and the way a person actually identifies are not congruent. For example, in the case of a bi-racial person who identifies as Black but visually presents as White, implicit biases may come into effect only after the person holding the bias encounters the information of how the person identifies racially.[47] There are circumstances in which the brain, once the person's racial identity is revealed, ascribes stereotypical traits of a Black person to the person. More likely, however, interpersonal exchanges result in a mix of vague unconscious complexities when the brain sees and responds as it would for a White person with some moments when the brain inconsistently ascribes attributes of Black stereotypes onto the now racialized person.[48]

This visibility and self-reporting of identity is key to better understanding how implicit bias affects the way one processes information and responds to the world and the people around them. It is also an attempt to clarify why the examples I have chosen focus on visible markers of identity and how those markers may be entirely inaccurate. Yet, still the implicit assumptions of what the observer thinks about a person, the implicit

Introduction 29

biases operating relating to the person being observed still apply, as if the assumptions carried by the observer are a reality.

This means that biases in dance education have the potential to inflict harm on marginalized or stigmatized colleagues, potential hires, and students alike, in a creative medium very much associated with visual and embodied experiences of those who dance, visual markers of bodies, behaviors, and written work of those who dance. When interacting with a dancer who does not meet a teacher's expectations of body size and has a fuller build, for example, implicit biases may cause undo negative interactions and unearned critical evaluative feedback about their health or performance.[49] When considering a new hire with a physical disability during a hiring process, biases about the capabilities of the candidate to meet the needs of the presumed majority, able-bodied students may inaccurately cause the search committee to exclude the candidate as unable to be successful in meeting job requirements.[50] During the evaluative process of a dancer's teaching, biases about gender and the dancer's ability to conform to gender expectations may negatively affect student evaluations of the dancer's teaching style, while the evaluator of the student evaluations may have a bias that skews toward statistical data as the whole truth instead of considering the implicit biases of the students.[51] Later on in this book there is further discussion of how implicit biases manifest along less defined social strata and more along personal, individual in-group/out-group circumstances. For the moment, I will focus on those biases that relate to systemic oppression to better establish the connection between implicit biases and their effects in dance education settings.

1

Privilege, Power, and Positionality
The Myth of Equality

These brain glitches, which I discussed in the last chapter as implicit biases, are part of a larger cycle that involves the participation of individuals but also extends far beyond the reach of one person in its ripple effects in the world. As I pointed out in the previous chapter, socialization is a key component in how implicit biases are formed. When implicit bias plays a role in prejudice or stereotyping a group of people, part of the equation involves the caste-like hierarchy of oppression. This cycle, **the cycle of oppression**,[1] is the unending, self-perpetuating subjugation of people by another group through the unjust use of power on a large scale.[2] The cycle of oppression is a way to understand how oppression is established and maintained at a societal level, and how individual actions, habits, and beliefs sustain this cycle. In this cycle, there are specific groups that receive privileges and advantages based solely on aspects of their identity. Some aspects of identity—whether these be socioeconomic status, race, gender, ability, sexuality, or physical size—afford these groups the social assumption of positive characteristics. In effect, under this system, privileged groups are given social power and privilege that other groups do not have access to.

The image of a cycle is a valuable model for understanding oppression because any stage in the cycle is an applicable starting point to understand how the system of oppression functions. The cycle is also self-sustaining, feeding and supporting itself. To better illuminate the effects of implicit bias and its role in the cycle of oppression, I will use these unconscious glitches that exist in the human brain-body as my starting point in the cycle throughout this book. The implicit biases socially held for specific groups of people, whether they be positive or negative, can feed the cycle's oppressive goals.

Remember, implicit biases exist in the brain-body because the brain-body has been fed a series of images, experiences, learned behaviors, and discussions that have created a pattern of anticipated value or inferiority. These experiences are collectively logged in the unconscious and express themselves as implicit bias. Biases are fed by messages based on insider-outsider cultures of marginalization and domination that are discussed in more detail in Chapter 2. This insider-outsider perspective is an approach to understanding societal structure that hinges on there being a hierarchy of groups of people in society. Insider groups have access to power and privileges, and outsiders are not afforded access to those powers and privileges. This is an approach to social order that hinges on there being a hierarchy of groups of people in society, with some insider groups having access to power and privileges, while outsiders are not afforded access to the same power and privileges. These cultural messages about who belongs and who does not are points of misinformation. These messages prey on the social contempt, disregard and marginalization of stigmatized groups and the normalization and acceptance of those with privileges. The brain-body takes in this misinformation as experiences that result in fear of difference in people.[3]

I had to grapple with this myself in third grade. In my transition from a predominantly White private school into my first public school, I noticed I was fearful of fellow Black students. I remember my internal dialogue at how ridiculous that was, as my entire family was Black. The question that stuck with me until studying racism in adulthood is why I was fearful of the students whose skin looked like mine. I now understand that I was inundated with media and other messages in my earlier schooling and personal life that centered White people as the friendly standard, and Black people as suspect outliers. Lucky for me, I had family and friends that could disrupt the pull that U.S. socialization offered.

Stereotypes develop when these messages are repeated frequently in various cultural contexts over sustained periods of time. Societies begin to accept these messages as true, factual, common occurrences, or accepted norms. A *stereotype*, as defined by Sheri Schmidt, is "a preconceived or oversimplified generalization about an entire group of people without regard for their individual differences."[4] Whether stereotypes are complimentary or derogatory, they are still harmful, because they group people together and make assumptions about individuals. People belonging to stereotyped groups, then, are not seen as individuals but, rather, as representatives of the attributes a stereotype assigns to their group.

Because the misinformed messaging, inaccurate representations, or lack of representations of people from marginalized groups is pervasive throughout our culture, the messages generated by stereotypes reach both marginalized and dominant groups alike. Take, for example, an exchange I had with an African American first-year dance major in a modern technique class I was teaching. She was passionate about dance, speaking with such full exuberance and excitement when she shared her passion for it. Yet, when it came to improvisational prompts inside the modern dance class, she was disengaged and did not fully commit to executing her movement choices in the class. An opportunity presented itself during the class improvisation for me to speak discreetly. I asked her why she wasn't committing fully to her movement. She responded that she just wasn't feeling the music we were dancing to.

This response crystalized for me the cultural context of the instruction I was providing. For this student, who shared that her passion for dance blossomed through dance forms like hip hop, this class was a new cultural context. The choice to use a live musician, who had no background in the musical genres this student was inspired by, to accompany the class was a culturally specific choice based on my indoctrination into cultural norms in the modern dance classes I was trained in. There was no real reason there could not have been different musical options offered for improvisational exploration during the class. This choice to blindly maintain the musical choices of the predominantly White spaces in which my training took place distanced this student from the norms she was accustomed to. But it was an unconscious choice of mine to associate the kinds of music I chose with this type of modern dance class until she brought it to my attention.

I had normalized the messaging about which musical styles are and are not acceptable for the modern dance classes I had experienced in my own training. I then expressed this bias with little to no thought about the relatively myopic experiences of what improvisational environments could sound like in the classes that I taught. Without this student sharing her own experience, I may have missed this opportunity to interrogate my biases on musical choice in modern dance classes. Without my understanding of the dominant cultural assumptions that structured the dance classes I grew up taking, I would not have been able to identify the bias expressed by the standards of what type of music is traditionally "appropriate" for modern dance class. I would not have been able to bring into conscious awareness how I centered predominantly White musical environments for improvisation, minimized musical environments from other cultures that were developed to support different types of improvisational dance spaces.

Vincent Thomas is one example of a dance educator who is able to see and address this issue of cultural inclusion and variation of musical genres in dance classes, who I was fortunate enough to take a class from. During the improvisational exploration of elements from the Laban Movement Analysis system,[5] Professor Thomas collaborated with a Black-bodied percussionist well-versed in vocal percussion to accompany the class. Replicating the percussive vocal techniques employed in hip hop to create the auditory experiential environment through which we were exploring these movement concepts was a powerful demonstration of cultural possibilities for artistry, inspiration, and exploration that I had not considered nor had access to previously in my movement training. The experience was profound and felt intentionally inclusive as it exposed me and others in the class to acoustic possibilities that were not tied to predominantly White musical genres. Professor Thomas's accompaniment choice demonstrated how different acoustic traditions are still tied to creating improvisational movement experiences. This inclusion of vocal percussion was referentially connected to hip hop, an underrepresented music genre in the context of movement improvisation in academic spaces. Furthermore, by incorporating the vocal percussion employed in the hip-hop musical tradition, this musical selection liberated hip hop from cultural stereotypes or social hierarchies of where this type of music *belongs* and where it does not.

Experiences like the one in Professor Thomas' workshop and my interaction with my own student have helped me to understand, become cognizant of, and process the ways that the stereotypes I was socialized with about hip hop and modern dance studio spaces were unfounded and needed deeper examination. These experiences helped me to understand that the genre of hip hop music and culture that I personally love and grew up listening to is not only appropriate for predominantly Black cultural spaces that are frequently marginalized and secluded so as to remain safe from the prying eyes of the forces of cultural appropriation and judgmental or dismissive outsiders. There was space for Black culture to be represented, engaged with, and respected for its valuable contributions to American creative invention, inspiration, and artistry by Black people in modern dance spaces. In addition, this experience helped me understand my inaccurate assumption that only predominantly White musical genres belong in modern dance class as creative inspiration and contributions.

The discovery of this assumption about music in modern dance classes in my own life also provides a window into how the next element of oppression takes hold in dance education. When stereotypes are so ubiquitous and long-standing, a byproduct is **internalized oppression**. This *internalized oppression* occurs when marginalized groups begin to believe they are inferior in the ways that stereotypes assert. ***Self-directed stigma*** may then occur wherein a person begins to make decisions navigating the world that are consistent with the oppressive biases they have encountered, essentially enacting those biases on themselves and others of the relevant identity marker. Conversely, dominant groups experience **internalized dominance**. In this situation, members of the dominant group begin to believe they are superior in the ways that stereotypes claim. In the above example, my inclination that hip hop music was somehow inappropriate for modern dance class is an example of internalized oppression I gained through lived experiences that told me hip hop is not *for* modern dance class. It is music relegated to the social or popular dance forms that are less attended to in the majority of higher education dance curriculum. An example of internalized dominance would be a person from a dominant group, in the case of race, a White person, perpetuating the idea that hip hop music is not an appropriate choice for modern dance classes, that it should only be relegated to hip hop dance classes, or that it should be superficially dropped into classes with little knowledge of the genre, history, or culture of the form as some sort of quick fix for cultural diversity and inclusion.

When generalizations about groups of people are believed by both marginalized and dominant groups, these generalizations become a collective bias. Whether conscious or unconscious, such biases result in unfounded assumptions or judgments, called **prejudices**. Prejudging an individual based upon their visible identity markers or cultural groups is harmful because it impedes the full consideration of the merits, talents, character, or disposition of the person as an individual. This leads to inaccurate judgments about people. As a result, innocence, knowledge, and goodness are assigned to some who are corrupt, for example, and depravity, suspicion, and ignorance ascribed to some who are upstanding members of society. In this current historical moment in the U.S., we see the veil being pulled back that protects police officers who are corrupt and villainizes Black people upon whom depraved cops inflict unconscionable and excessive violence. By way of mobile phone video cameras in the hands of bystanders capturing these interactions all over the country, the U.S. has been inundated with new, lived experiences to be stored as implicit memories. These new video recordings are disrupting the prejudices that police enforcement are usually innocent, and Black people are usually guilty.

These prejudices are then enacted through **discrimination** in ways that result in unfounded decisions on whether to accept and celebrate or reject and castigate a person. Sensoy and DiAngelo define *discrimination* as "action based on prejudices toward social others. How we *think* about social groups of people determines how we *act* toward them."[6] Discrimination presents itself in two ways: (1) in favor of a person based on prejudices that privilege them or (2) in opposition to a person based on prejudices that disadvantage them. In dance education discrimination may look like (1) the decision to accept a student into a class or a program who do not meet standards, but due to prejudicial logics are determined to be acceptable, or (2) the decision to deny a student access to opportunities and resources when, outside prejudicial actions, that student would otherwise be afforded access just like everyone else. These discriminatory factors based on prejudicial stereotypes shape deliberations that should be based on evidence and the equitable evaluation of each individual. These discriminatory dispositions can present in a number of ways in a dance program. It can be present in the evaluation and assessment of students, the selection of students for various opportunities or awards, auditions and acceptance for those programs that require auditions to enroll in the program, and in the hiring, evaluation, or promotion of teachers.

While individuals can discriminate against other individuals, this is also a method that organizations, businesses, and institutions integrate into explicit policies or unspoken standards that result in oppressive and discriminatory patterns of decision-making and behaviors within their institutional culture. This communal, organized group of dance educators can include private dance studios, Pre-Kindergarten–12th grade (PK-12) schools, higher education dance programs, and supporting non-profit or municipal dance class programming. When institutions use these inaccurate assumptions to judge groups of people, it perpetuates and enforces falsehoods as normal practices in the culture of the organization. This results in **institutionalized oppression**. Sheri Schmidt defines *institutionalized oppression* as "the systematic subjugation of a group of people by another group of people with access to social power, the result of which benefits one group over the other and is maintained by social beliefs and practices."[7] Institutionalized oppression, then, takes place when the discrimination becomes integral to how protocols, policies, and determinations are established in decision-making and behaviors in an institution or across institutions.

For example, there is a misconception that ballet is the foundation of all dance forms—a common myth perpetuated in media content in the U.S. This assumption is, in turn, articulated in dance program practices by way of requiring ballet training for students in order for them to be accepted into a dance program. This example of institutionalized oppression is also a common dance program requirement in higher education institutions: ballet or modern dance classes are often required in order to graduate. Requiring these specific kinds of dance practices centers Western concert dance forms—ballet and modern dance—as the standard or acceptable mode of dance that should be learned in order to attain a degree in dance. This is the result of historical stereotypes of ballet and modern dance being the quintessential forms that, in the societal hierarchy of dance forms, are most valued by those in dominant positions in the dance community.

While it may seem that the dance forms that were first developed in the U.S., such as hip hop, Appalachian clogging, Swing dance, or Chicago Stepping, to name a few, would be the most logical dance forms around which to center a U.S. dance curriculum or at least be considered Western dance forms, these forms are not required by and large across dance programs and are not categorized as Western dance forms.[8] Outside of modern dance, dance forms born from U.S. culture, if present at all in the curriculum, more often serve as supplemental, optional courses for students. Ballet, a form originating in Europe, and modern dance, a form with its roots in the U.S. and Europe, are the forms more often required in a majority of exclusive, audition-based dance programs. This is an example of institutional oppression that centers predominantly White concert dance forms as dominant and central in dance education and assigning other dance forms developed in the U.S. to the margins of programming and affording those non–White dancers who participate in these forms benefits for doing so.

The result of the ubiquity and dominance of ballet and modern dance in educational programs is that forms that are not considered the White, upper class forms of Western concert dance, are programmatically marginalized, with less prospects for lasting, full-time positions specializing in these forms and a lack of in-depth study dedicated to these forms in higher education institutions. While regional variations may apply, this is also an element in a number of PK-12 educational institutions and studios across the U.S. Students in private dance studios or primary and secondary education programs often need to have access to ballet and/or modern dance forms in order to be strong candidates for a number of higher education institutions. These candidates then graduate from undergraduate programs with a greater level of access to training and opportunities to work with professionals in the field of concert dance through their dance program education. Training and access to the field of professional concert dance affords those trained in ballet and modern dance access to funding opportunities to participate in dance companies and other professional opportunities. With the significant exception of commercial dance opportunities,[9] this leaves little room for dance forms that do not fall under the label of Western concert dance in the way of funding opportunities, training, and access to economically sustaining career opportunities.

With the dominance and ubiquity of modern and ballet as central forms for educational advancement in the field of dance education, academic institutions have perpetuated a need for students to be, open to learning or exposed to, at minimum, and be proficient, at most, in modern and ballet in order for them to be successful, admitted to, or hirable in dance education settings. Those that do not have proficiency in at least one of these two forms are often positioned as marginalized, novelty, temporary members of the dance education field.[10] When this problem becomes apparent across a number of organizations and institutions as students progress through their education and training as dancers, it is challenging to counter the floodgates of privileges that accrue to modern dance and ballet as genres that do not apply in comprehensive ways to other dance genres. In this way the system is unbalanced. It affords benefits to those who have the interest and financial capacity to study ballet and modern dance, and does not often benefit those who have not trained in these forms of dance. These dance genres are now institutionalized in their privileges and position of power in the field of dance education.

The message about the significance of ballet and modern dance in dance education becomes not just a few people who have this opinion, but rather, a system of various programs, organizations, and gatekeeping educators and administrators who reinforce this idea. At this point the idea that ballet and modern dance are needed to thrive become pervasive across systems of dance education, not just individual opinions of dance educators and administrators. It means that an individual no longer has to have a personal opinion about the importance of ballet or modern dance. Even if they did, it would not change the mounting access and privileges these dance forms convey to students. The idea of ballet and modern dance being central and necessary in dance education curricula is no longer personal to individuals but a systemic environment that individual educators who want to see their students succeed in dance education feel they must be knowledgeable about and responsive to.

ACTIVITY BOX #3: What If Dance...

What would the field of dance education look like if dancers who had a passion for other forms of dance were able to establish the value of those forms as adding as much value to understanding the moving, expressive body as ballet and modern dance? What would it look like if dancers with expertise in these other forms were able to establish programs from PK-12 to higher education that centered study in that form? How might the examples of dance shown in various dance classes look if taught by instructors with a bias and expertise in dance forms other than ballet and modern dance? How might student experience change if instructors who had biases for other forms were hired and encouraged to share how they understand dance based on biases that represent their cultural moorings?

1. Privilege, Power, and Positionality

What might community engagement look like in dance classes, performances, and programs if there was a bias for different dance forms than ballet and modern dance?

In this moment of the cycle, it becomes apparent that there is a difference between the general definition of oppression on an individual scale and how it is activated in the context of societal injustices. **Oppression** consists of the combination of aforementioned prejudice and discrimination that is then coupled with institutional powers and systems that uphold these prejudices and discrimination. This is the distinction between systemic oppression and the bigotry and hatred for another person because of their social group status. Systemic oppression does not require a personal feeling or sentiment for those being oppressed. The protocols, policies, and values in dance education programming across the U.S. dictate whether a person will be accepted or denied whether individual educators or administrators personally like a student or not. Because of the systemic factors of dominant culture at play, to have a hatred for the dance forms of ballet or modern dance, for example, may be a personal bias wherein an individual, or even a dance program may discriminate against those who have a ballet or modern dance background. But in the larger society, the systemic structures of dance education in the U.S. benefit ballet and modern dance as genres on a larger more pervasive scale that is difficult to subvert or escape living in the U.S.

A person from a marginalized group, in this example a cultural insider from a marginalized dance form, carries biases, as everyone is exposed to implicit memories, and can therefore have prejudices against others. However, marginalized groups—in this case, those cultural insiders of marginalized dance forms—are not afforded power to create policies, determine who is included or excluded in social groups or institutions, or enforce these prejudices in ways that are socially pervasive across the dance education institutions in the U.S. While bigotry and prejudice are certainly attributes that individuals can carry and express whether they are part of marginalized groups or dominant groups, it is only the members of the dominant group—in this case, cultural insiders of the predominantly White concert dance forms, ballet and modern dance—that have the access to larger systems, such as the economic successes of private dance studios, academic privileges of majority stakeholders in tenured faculty positions, major dance media publications, state and federal advocacy platforms, and dance funding institutions, to enact inclusion or exclusion of others across the field of dance education.

Access to power within these systems supports and validates the dominant group's perspectives and prejudices, and, as such, those perspectives are structured into the systems and cultures of the institutions. In the case of educational institutions, individual actors include administrators, staff, board members, and educators who manage, enforce, and advise on policy. Because the power and privilege I am tracking in the field of dance education is one of the predominantly White, upper class educational staples of ballet and modern dance, those who study or have aesthetic biases towards those genres attain privileges in the field that sustain these dance genres as the predominant forms in the field of dance education.

Of course, there is certainly a more complex dynamic as we consider intersections of other identity markers like race, gender, sexuality, socioeconomic class, body size, and ability. Any given individual holds both dominant and minoritized aspects of their identity. For example, a ballet dancer may have the socially dominant aspects of their identity of being White-bodied (physically presenting as White), physically able-bodied, and a U.S. citizen. At the same time this same person, may be a female-identifying, biracial self-identifying Black person, from a lower socioeconomic status, with a cognitive disability unseen to those who watch the person dance. This means that while the value and centrality of ballet and modern dance for this dancer are reified in dance education systems through this power dynamic, individuals that carry marginalized statuses such as physical disabilities or Black, Indigenous, and people of color (BIPOC) identities, do not receive an equal amount of power and access as White, able-bodied ballet and modern dancers receive.

Access to ballet and modern dance do still afford some level of access and privilege to marginalized groups in the U.S. system of dance education through mechanisms that reify power structures. In public school education this includes local, state, and federal politicians and their voting constituents who fund education and make policies. At privately-owned schools, organizations, and studios, the funders, whether they be paying clients or philanthropists, have a significant influence on institutional decisions. All of these players must carry forward with some familiarity with at least, and some bias toward at most, the genres of ballet and modern dance in dance education.

As marginalized groups are denied access and/or fed messages they are not entitled to resources, opportunities, and privileges that the dominant groups benefit from, the results are often devastating in systemic ways. The oppression that manifests through the largest systems that organize society is comprehensive in ways that encourage the internalization of feelings of entitlement and superiority on behalf of the dominant groups and feelings of restriction and disregard for marginalized groups.

1. Privilege, Power, and Positionality   41

The list of internalized factors of socioeconomic power dynamics and oppression is long, as these biases inform decisions made by individuals in every aspect of life from the microcosm of who we gravitate to as artists, to the macrocosm of how dance education sites sustain themselves. So pervasive are the effects systemic injustices and oppression have on the status, behavior, and successes (or lack thereof) of marginalized people, that dominant groups then tend to use this "evidence" as reason to be insensitive, unsympathetic, or unsupportive of the plight of the marginalized groups. Robin DiAngelo articulates this clearly:

> Oppression becomes justified in large part based upon the impact that generations of oppression has had on the minoritized group. Long-term systematic oppression in access to resources, social acceptance, housing, education, employment, health care, and economic development has devastating effects. Due to generations of being denied full access to the resources of society, the minoritized group occupies a much lower overall position. The minoritized group must develop survival strategies in order to cope with long-term oppression. Many of these patterns will be empowering to the minoritized group, but some of these patterns will not be healthy and will not support their survival. For example, there may be increased drug and alcohol use, or increased rates of suicide. The dominant group uses the position and patterns of the minoritized group to rationalize the oppression and blame the minoritized group for its condition, attributing the effects of historical oppression to the lack of a work ethic, personal, cultural or family values, biology, or an element in their genetic makeup. Thus, the dominant group justifies the oppression of the minoritized group *based on the effects of having oppressed them*.[11]

Such effects of oppression are used to justify the further disenfranchisement of marginalized people. This errant justification thus heightens the internalized oppression of marginalized groups and the internalized dominance of dominant groups.

The implicit memories of oppression's inequities then serve to justify oppression and reify implicit biases. This is where implicit biases can be both activated, i.e., experienced for the first time and substantiated, and simultaneously evidenced as data that existing biases are true. Without pervasive messages that simultaneously stigmatize marginalized groups and generate the misinformed justification of why some groups are marginalized, invisible, or unimportant, the cycle of oppression does not have roots from which to grow. Robin James articulates this by explaining that "the systematic account of privilege and oppression treats individual people as necessary, but not sufficient, causes of social inequality."[12] The common justification for inequities does not hold without the socially pervasive messages about differences between groups of people in society and the specious values or deficits of those groups. These pervasive messages that stigmatize oppressed groups create the implicit memories upon which implicit biases against these groups are sustained.

ACTIVITY BOX #4: Power by the Numbers

Having all students wear a number that they cannot see but can be seen by others. The number corresponds to their level of importance in the room. For example, the person wearing the number one is ascribed the most importance while the person wearing the number thirty in a classroom of thirty students is ascribed the least importance. Then the instructor assigns a group planning activity where students have to interact with each other based on their ascribed number and corresponding level of importance. The group activity can be any activity that requires students to communicate, brainstorm ideas, and make decisions such as planning a party or event or even creating a small movement phrase.

After students complete that activity, students take off their numbers to see what numbers they had. Then students reflect on what happened and how they felt while engaging in the activity. If there is time, I sometimes supplement this activity with video clips about inequity or how implicit bias affects our interactions with one another to help illuminate this process, what to look for in identifying it, and how to disrupt these habits in working with each other.

෴

Socialization: In-Group/Out-Group Orientation in Dance

Social hierarchies are part of U.S. social conditioning and one of the most significant factors that feeds biases both explicit and implicit. Those raised in the U.S., unless raised in a very insular setting intentionally removed from hierarchical structures and messaging, are socialized to think of their relationship to others in an in-group/out-group stratum of class and popularity that relies on social identifiers such as race, socioeconomic class, ability, body size or shape, etc. These hierarchies are ingrained in such a way that, in looking at some common structures as binary, it would be a very quick sorting of which of the two categories is dominant or in-group and which is marginalized or out-group. See how quickly you can sort through the following chart:

1. Privilege, Power, and Positionality

Poor	Wealthy
Tall	Short
Gender binary	Gender fluidity/continuum
White	Indigenous
U.S. citizen	U.S. resident
Abled	Disabled
Thick-bodied	Thin-bodied
Brain/Intellect/Ideas	Body/Behavior/Action

Even if you consider yourself a person who is inclusive and does not believe in these binary divisions or in the inequity of these social categories, it is still possible to determine which of each binary in U.S. society are considered dominant, centered, the norm, or standard. The ability to quickly make such a determination stems from the implicit memories, lived experiences, and often-passive and unintended messages one is exposed to living in the U.S. This socialization affects our preferences, likes, and dislikes. These messages are carried around in our implicit memories and influence what a person *should* want to be associated with or estranged from, and even what a person *should* like or dislike. This is the context in which the field of dance and, by extension, dance education lives.

Aesthetics is what is perceived or accepted as beautiful. It is through these power-laden messages about aesthetic standards that those who are not a part of a privileged community can benefit by believing in the same standards of the dominant groups and/or by embodying those standards. Robin James provides an example of this relationship between the power structures of a society and aesthetics.[13] James explains this as follows:

> While white people or straight men do benefit from white heteropatriarchy, participation in white heteropatriarchy is not limited to straight white men. For example, women who buy into patriarchy can still secondarily or indirectly benefit from patriarchy: women who enforce patriarchal beauty standards are often rewarded with male attention, higher salaries, etc.[14]

In the dance world, this participation in a heteropatriarchal aesthetic may involve ideas such as assigning only male-identifying dancers roles in which they lift female-identifying dancers, a long-enforced heteronormative notion that men are strong and thus do the lifting based on gender, not necessarily strength. This then becomes an aesthetic choice that reinforces the *masculine = strong* social message. Taking into consideration the ways in which societal influence informs how a member of the society perceives, evaluates, and organizes their understanding of the world, aesthetics and what is beautiful is a pertinent aspect to be considered in the field of dance education.

Privilege, for James, is conveyed to those who ascribe to the messages about social hierarchy. This benefit of privileges is bestowed based on the larger systemic messages such as those displayed in the chart above no matter whether you are in the dominant status or not. When an individual aligns with and replicates the messages of social hierarchy, the system affords those individuals access and acceptance to societal privileges such as acknowledgment in the way of awards or grants in dance; employment as dancer or dance educator; and gatekeeping status as dance adjudicators, dance education administrators, board members for arts organizations, or dance selection panelists. Often, James argues, discriminatory behavior or stereotyping others is often errantly perceived as an individual's flaw instead of a systemic structure within which the individual exists, whether intentionally or passively, consciously, or unconsciously. The same can be said of marginalized members who have internalized the negative stereotypes and assumptions society replicates about them as true. Neither of these are individual deficits, but rather reflections of the hierarchical socialization process.

If you are a marginalized member of the dance community that performs a deference and appreciation to dominant members of the community when granted an earned opportunity, there is benefit for maintaining the social expectations of hierarchical roles. The expectation being that if you are of a socially lower rank, you should show appreciation to more dominant members for opportunities that structurally would not have been afforded to you due to systematic discrimination. If you are a dominant group member who does not take pity on marginalized community members, but rather asserts that they should be respected, honored, and accepted under institutional standards and qualifications as equals in the community because of their earned talent, creative work, and/or intellect, this is divergent from the social hierarchy structures of the U.S. The expectation being that, as a dominant group member, your role is to serve as gatekeeper and savior that allows and extends the unexpected favor of accepting the lower ranking community member into the institution. If your creative work is not a Western concert dance form, but references some aspect of the Western concert dance canon, your work may be considered in selection processes, in part, because of its connection to the established norms and standards of the social dominance hierarchy of the U.S.

The effects of implicit bias function in that unconscious, systemic way where the dominant groups in society bestow privileges to those that support, participate in, and contribute to messages that bolster the social dominance hierarchy and can then mask the social dynamics of the decision by calling it aesthetic evaluation—how well-crafted, unique, innovative, creative the dancer or choreographer's voice in the field of dance is purported to be. In the case of a dance organization deciding what dance work will be selected for a performance season, those bestowed with the power to determine who will be selected are examining aspects of aesthetics, creative vision, and voice. What James asserts is that organizations that align with U.S. societal systems of hierarchy are looking for dances that are consistent with the standards set forth by U.S. social norms. The selection process then has as much to do with the social expectations of what dance works are expected to be valued in the aesthetics of the U.S. as it does with each individual artist.

An anecdotal way I illustrate the connection between aesthetic preferences and identity in my classes is by discussing our assumptions about why people who like hip hop music don't like country music. In my workshops, when I share this example students who grew up in the U.S. never request a further explanation of my claim. There is an implicit understanding about these genres of music and their audiences that is effectively coded into our culture. A similar point can be made within the field of dance. Of course, there are individuals that might love both hip hop dance and classical ballet or country line dancing. But there are messages about identity, class, and culture baked into these aesthetic preferences that so often signal what *type* of person you are. In this structure, individuals are both products of a system that enacts societal paradigms on them and also actors within that very same paradigm who carry forward, replicate, or are in relationship with those societal structures no matter the intent of an individual's personal aesthetic preferences. This is why individual people are not the sole cause of inequity, but, rather, a necessary carrier of inequity. At the same time by naming inequities and implicit biases as they manifest, individuals can also be a potential part of equitable solutions to societal issues.

The messages and underlying assumptions that organize how information is framed even affects how we think we learn what we know. With mandatory public education being a central aspect of U.S. culture, many have been socialized to believe that the methods usually employed in formal school settings—such as tests, lectures, and reading—are how the human brain-body learns. While tests, lectures, and reading may constitute some of the ways people evidence learning, many other learning mechanisms are left largely underrepresented or invisible—such as embodied learning, to name one many dance educators are familiar with. This has been well-documented in research on the "hidden curriculum," which cites the positive effects of embodied learning while acknowledging its underrepresentation in pedagogy.[15] There has been a significant gap in utilization and research of embodied learning practices in PK-12 education due to the long history of a bias toward mental techniques of student learning.[16] The Cartesian split between the thinking brain and profane body continues in discussions in the field of dance education, as well as later on in this book when I consider the effects of implicit bias in studio and classroom instruction.[17]

Socialization includes "messages, beliefs, images, associations, internalized superiority [or inferiority] and entitlement [or disenfranchisement/subordination], perceptions, and emotions."[18] The socialization process is both an individual process and a collective one that takes place in the cultures and communities of which we are a part. This process of learning to understand how social interaction works is how we establish which societal groups we are a part of—our nation, our ethnicity, our family, etc.—and which groups we stand apart from. For example, I identify myself as a modern dancer generally, and as a postmodern subgroup member of the modern dance community based on my dance education experience. However, as an African American, I identify with the dances of early hip hop based on my cultural background even though I do not consider myself a hip hop dancer by profession. In this way socialization is complex, and an individual can be a member of various groups based on the communities they belong to. But the tendency to group people results in stereotypes and prejudices of groups, both ones we may identify with and those we may not. Even though I have a more developed professional background in postmodern dance, it is not uncommon for people who do not know my dance background to ask me about Alvin Ailey, hip hop, or West African dance, all forms associated with Black culture. Discrimination results from these stereotypes and prejudices when the person who maintains stereotypes and prejudices as truths have the power to include, exclude, or evaluate individuals or groups of people based on those stereotypes and prejudices. Even before discrimination manifests overtly, discriminatory harm can be felt in seemingly innocuous contexts. I once had a three-year old tell me that men do not eat salads, as if he were cueing me in on a bit of useful wisdom he had garnered. His life experiences not only conditioned him to think of gender as a binary construct, but also to internalize the observed behaviors of people and/or statements made by those around him into what he thought of as obvious fact.

The brain's compulsion to find connections and patterns, to differentiate one thing from another, to group what it perceives as similar items together, and to abstract discrete experiences, objects, or people into large general categories is also how biases and stereotypes are birthed. The human brain begins to correlate behaviors or characteristics with groups of people. While some of this process is self-directed, much of it is internalized via socialization—the behaviors and assumptions enacted by others around us—whether it be our family members or friends during childhood, teachers in school, media content, or neighbors and community members.

When predetermined sociocultural categories are taught to and experienced by children, these categories become foundational to how that child perceives the world. The process of differentiating visual markers of boy from girl, or Black from White from Asian start at very early ages and are guided by social constructs of the distinctions between these categories.[19] Now that some children in the U.S. are receiving new messaging—how gender can be understood as a continuum rather than a binary, for example—the differentiation process will be different for them than it was for me growing up.

Predetermined sociocultural categories affect the way humans view the world and organize knowledge. These categories act as operators that activate before we have any interaction with an individual. These assumptive categorizations can lead to body prejudice or misinterpreting the meaning of movement behaviors based on generalizations linked to the observer's socialization and cultural perspective.[20] The physical example I often use of the body prejudices in a dance studio setting is to saunter past the class with an extreme swayback posture with my sternum leading, asking students to call out what they assume about a person who walks this way. Students call out a number of different assumptions, with common assignations of sexually assertive or low class. Then I walk across the room with my chest sunken back and my pelvis leading with my weight back in my heels. Students often assign qualities of lazy or laid back to this walking posture. These physical demonstrations that trigger character correlations from students help illustrate for students how quickly prejudices can affect how we think about a person.

Even when there is no decision-making or evaluative power for the person carrying unpacked stereotypes or prejudices, **microaggressions** can still occur. In the earlier example of the young boy who assumed men don't eat salads, what then of the fellow three-year old boy or queer classmate who loves to eat salad sitting in earshot of this exchange? Derald Wing Sue defines *microaggressions* as "the brief and commonplace daily verbal, behavioral, and environmental indignities, whether intentional or unintentional, that communicate hostile, derogatory, or negative racial, gender, sexual-orientation, and religious slights and insults to the target person or group."[21] A physical microaggression could be a White person pulling their bag closer to them when passing a Black-bodied person. This microaggression is based on the stereotype that Black people are criminals and results in the White person attempting to secure their bag in anticipation of the Black-bodied person taking the bag. Asking the one BIPOC person in a group of White people where their family is from is a verbal microaggression. This verbal microaggression is based on the stereotype that BIPOC people are not originally from the U.S. In effect, biases can result in stereotypical assumptions that then manifest in these behavioral or verbal microaggressions whether that harm is intentional or not.

ACTIVITY BOX #5: Combs and Kangaroos

To disrupt and explore what it is like to step outside of pre-established social categories, I offer the following activity. Bring into the class three intentionally random and seemingly unrelated items. Challenge students to list as many ways the items are related or what they have in common as they can think up. Students then share their lists, crossing off any ideas that have already been shared with others.

Remember the frame of this activity is to remember that things that may seem very disconnected, with creativity, can be related in unexpected ways. As it is developmentally appropriate, also share that the reasons we know to arrange how things are related is because we have been exposed to educational systems and other life experiences that have taught us pre-determined frames with which to categorize things. You may then want to challenge the class to invest in finding new categories for ideas or objects for the duration of the class term. Reflect on the following statement: *We are thinking outside of those boxes we already know into new creative possibilities.* This activity can then connect to the decision-making or creative processes throughout the class.

In the case of systemic social categories, the knowledge constituted from the U.S. systems of oppression, and also the U.S. system's corresponding aesthetic standards are organized via ideas of right and wrong and the greater societal good or rank. Thus, aesthetics are the social measure of what we think is good and beautiful, relying on the messages disseminated through social systems. Aesthetics are, therefore, an element of why the effects of the cycle of oppression are pervasive. The lack of awareness of the connection between aesthetics and oppression is why messages about standards of beauty are seemingly so harmless and individual. Oppressive messages are sustained by the leisure elements of entertainment, fashion, beauty, and the arts.[22] These aspects of society are implicit memory makers, a mass-production method of repeatedly relaying messages in ways that seem innocuous in our leisure and entertainment experiences. However, the cumulative effect is that baselines of normativity are established, determining what is attractive, perverse, conventional, funny, and exotic. Aesthetic standards are another way to both promote and enforce what is deemed valuable or powerful in a culture and what is not via mechanisms where critical examination and accountability are not at the forefront for the mass audience.

Cultural **hegemony**, meaning the common-sense elements a society, culture, or nation takes as obvious and overriding evidence of truth, is another way to articulate or engage with this messaging that is ubiquitous in a society.[23] There was a long period of time in my early life and dance training that the erroneous statement I mentioned before of ballet being the foundation of all dance would have seemed to be an "obvious truth" of dance rather than a myopic perspective on dance. The concept of hegemony is a way to describe the inundation of cultural messaging that results in norms borne out by implicit bias. When a society, for example, is inundated with images of thin women associated with beauty, health, power, wealth, attention, and agency, while thicker, fuller bodied women are shown in advertisements, entertainment content, and health segments as less attractive, unhealthy, impotent, comical, lower class, discounted, or incapable of self-control, the society's values about women's bodies and their relationship to power in that society are on full display. These societal signals reify social messages that thin women are the standard or the preferred aesthetic to strive for or celebrate in U.S. society. What often goes unnoticed in the arena of beauty and aesthetic sensibilities is its connection to systems of power.

Aesthetics both born from and also replicated through hegemony are a way in which systemic structures are maintained via omnipresent messages through various modes of artistic and entertainment platforms from internet content, to print advertisements, to concert stages. This hierarchical structure is then maintained by language and categorization such as popular (pop) art versus classical art and social or vernacular dance versus concert dance.[24] It is within these cordoned off branches of creative realizations that socioeconomic class and social divides are maintained through funding, ticket price, placement of advertisements based on intended audience, and access to reviewers. Through this maneuvering of what art gets seen where, at what price point, and by what audience and reviewers, societal messages that reify boundaries between types of viewers, or target audiences of that art are established. This further solidifies the everyday occurrence of what is hegemony—what is collectively experienced and understood to be "true" by the society. Even audiences that establish counter-narratives are in some level of relationship to these societal standards, making intentional choices of how to be in response to social norms and assumptions.

Thus, if Chicago Steppers, a social dance form growing out of African American communities in Chicago, were provided access to national grant funding, concert dance venues, and the critical reviews of well-established dance critics, they would be deemed a valuable aesthetic voice in the field of dance. But because the Chicago Steppers community does not have access or chooses not to engage in the institutions of "high art," but, instead, perform in dance halls within an insular cultural community not seeking external grant funding, the aesthetic standards of the dance form are not central to the stories of dance in the U.S. Modern dance and ballet continue to be centered genres in dance education, even though Chicago Stepping originated in the U.S. while modern (at least solely) and ballet did not.[25] These hegemonic forces center and value the predominantly White, upper class, exclusive ballet and modern dance forms in dance education and marginalize U.S. social dances. In this way in dance education valuing the dance forms associated with Whiteness, access to resources to train in a dance form, and upper-class socioeconomic status are normalized attitudes and behaviors that then become implicit biases and go unnoticed in their ubiquity.

Activity Box #6: Illogical Norms

I have posed a question of why the Chicago Steppers dance form isn't part of the U.S. dance canon in educational settings for dance even though it is a form developed in the U.S. Brainstorm other questions or examples of common knowledge or assumptions about dance that when sorted through logic do not quite make sense without signals from socialization. For example, what other dance forms created in the U.S. are not included in your current dance program or past dance training? What are some other examples of things in your dance education training that don't quite make sense in the community? Why do they seem illogical to you? Why do you think they exist as illogical factors in the dance education community? Have students share some of their examples with the class for discussion.

2

Social Markers of Bias

The implicit biases that are common to socialization in the U.S. create categories of oppression in dance education. For example, the *Project Implicit* Implicit Association Tests (IAT) currently has fifteen different categories of implicit bias options that a person can test for to discover what biases they may not know they have.[1] In social justice contexts, these biases are associated with various mechanisms of power and oppression. Below is a chart of some commonly-held sociocultural oppressions and corresponding discriminatory categories that are systemically enforced in the U.S. I have intentionally chosen the following list to highlight areas of marginalization that feel particularly pertinent in the field of dance. These categories are also linked to the normalized aesthetic sensibilities in the U.S. Note that the majority of these categories of marginalization are based in a binary orientation, which itself speaks to a bias held over from early philosophical orientations toward binary thinking.

Dominant	*Marginalized*	*Form of Oppression*
Male	Female	Sexism
White Race	non–White Races	Racism
Light-skinned	Dark-skinned	Colorism
Thin-bodied	Full-bodied	Sizeism
Heterosexual	Homosexual	Heterosexism
Able body	Disabled body	Ableism
Rich	Poor	Classism
Young	Old	Ageism

A number of these categories rely on visual representation, whether they are assumed to be apparent visibly (i.e., how someone is dressed may indicate markers of classism, heterosexism, etc.), or wholly determined based on visual markers (i.e., skin color and body shape resulting in colorism, sizeism, etc.). The visual field is part of the reason these issues and corresponding biases are so prevalent in the field of dance, a field based largely on aesthetics and visual representations of the moving, dancing body. For those elements listed that aren't solely dependent on visual bodily markers like skin color, there are cultural assumptions based on behavior associated with those elements as well. For example, in dance, a person with an invisible disability may not be marked as an outsider through visual markers like a person with a visible disability until behaviors or conversations with the dancer disclose this marginalized status.

When these social messages about identity markers are combined with a hierarchical orientation to society, a person perceives other individuals as having more or less power in social settings than they do. This social perspective is called **Social Dominance Orientation (SDO)** in social science research. SDO is an area of study that tracks a person's perception of society as a hierarchical construct. People who perceive the social environment through the lens of *Social Dominance Orientation (SDO)* see some people as more important than others.[2]

The aversion to obesity or larger bodies in dance reflects a socially dominant orientation to bodily size. Psychologists Kerry O'Brian, John Hunter, and Mike Banks assert "a growing body of research suggests that the negative health consequences associated with obesity may be attenuated by regular exercise, even in the absence of reductions in adiposity [obesity]."[3] Often dancers, choreographers, educators, and even medical professionals find it a commonplace notion that obese dancers are most likely physically unfit and, therefore, less able to fulfill the demands of the profession or find success in the field of dance. For those seeking in-group status in dance, it would benefit them in gaining and maintaining that physical weight and size status to be agreeable on this tenet, one that is, in this case, not just prevalent in the field of dance but also often supported by messaging about larger bodies generally in the U.S.

Commonly held beliefs about body size hold until events such as this encounter, which I had some decades ago, take place to call those beliefs into question. I had developed a friendly connection with a colleague in New York City who had recently moved to the city from the Catalonia region of Spain. She had performed postmodern and modern dance on concert stages in Europe for a number of years and had a classically thin, lean body. Her sternum was visible, as were the sinews of her muscles. We discussed where she might be able to take classes in the postmodern dance scene in New York City. I recommended some studios and teachers I particularly appreciated. The following week this colleague returned sharing her excitement about a particular class that she took, which was also one of my favorites to frequent. As I recollect the gist and sentiment of this exchange, I noticed she explained in a blunt and direct way that when she first entered the studio for class, she said to herself, "Oh my! This woman is fat. How will she be able to teach me, you know?" She continued with exasperated joy and delight at her pleasant surprise: "But then when I began the class, it was so difficult I was not able to finish the class. I mean, how is she able to do this, you know?"

Her joy at upending the assumptions about the teacher's body size undergirding the studio experience she shared was a wonderfully memorable moment for me. Not only did it connect us in our absolute joy and respect for the class as a stellar and challenging postmodern dance class, it also was an exuberant opening and challenging of what she knew and how she understood the dancing body to be. She was able to name and acknowledge her assumptions that the instructor would not be able to teach a challenging, valuable class because of her body size. It was a thrill to see her enjoy how wrong her assumptions were that a fuller-bodied dancer would not be able to be an effective dance teacher. There were skills this voluptuous, professional dancer carried with her and shared in her classes that disrupted what this colleague of mine relied on to move through the classwork. If it was not the slender facility of moving through the bones enveloped in the lean, lightness of this body from Catalonia, what was this curvy, robust body using to so eloquently and effortlessly articulate her body? Was it less about how much weight a dancer carried and more about the facile access to core support and bodily connectivity that resulted in a rigorous dance class? While it is a rarity to see fuller-bodied performers in ballet and modern dance, voluptuous bodies of the African diaspora often flawlessly execute high-impact, feats of cardiovascular exceptionalism, with no acknowledgment of the facility with which they activate their whole bodies in performances around the world. Unfortunately, the White woman who taught this postmodern dance class was not part of such a community of diverse sizes and shapes regularly performing modern dance, and was seen as an anomaly in the field of dance.

When there are notable examples of thicker-bodied dancers who excel in professional dance performances and choreographies, the question follows as to why anti-fat bias persists in the field of dance. These kinds of questions arise when an implicit belief or attitude is unsettled through an encounter with an event or example that runs counter to that belief. If there is a conscious awareness of this cognitive fracture, the brain-body has the capacity to restructure the belief to more accurately reflect the lived experience of the individual. More often, however, there is no conscious awareness that this process is taking place. As is so often the case, the brain-body then either categorizes the anomaly as an outlier to be held separate and apart from the fully intact commonly held belief, or else the outlier is incorporated into a different association in the mind that supports an altogether different disposition. For example, exposure to an exceptional, thicker dance performer may get integrated into memory and over time into our belief system as an institution being particularly inclusive and commendable for integrating such an anomalous performer into the fold rather than concluding that the performer is a disruptor of the unspoken assumption that successful dancers are thin.

In addition to the pervasive biases that reflect dominant culture across the country, there are also local or situational in-group/out-group dynamics that are not operational at the larger level of society. These biases operate in the local community, but are not necessarily prevalent in a broader sense. For example, does your local dance community support Black dancers wearing tights that resemble their skin tone, or wearing tights that are uniform to pink tights that more closely resemble the skin tones of White-bodied people? Does your dance program or dance community have any requirement for students to wear tights at all? The local community's approach to decisions such as this is significant in establishing a culture of who is an **in-group member** and who is an **out-group member**. *In-group members* are those members of the community that are dominant or favored in the community, especially by those in positions of power. *Out-group members* are members of the community that are stigmatized, marginalized, or unfavored in the community, especially by those in positions of power. Furthermore, according to research in group socialization and social identity, when individuals perceive themselves to be a member of the in-group of a social group, they are more likely to hold negative biases against those they perceive to be out-group members of the relevant group.[4]

Activity Box #7: Local or Larger

Brainstorm some biases you know of in dance. These could be your own personal biases, biases you have heard from others, or biases you have seen or experienced beyond a personal exchange between people, like on tv or social media. Categorize what biases you think are local and would not apply outside of a specific group of people in the U.S. and what biases you think would apply in most situations across the U.S. For the list of local biases you feel are only common within a specific group, what do you feel holds these group members together or establishes them as distinct from the broader U.S. group identification? Remember to include some of your own biases that are group-specific and biases you hold that you think are more prominent across the U.S. For an additional option, are there international biases you can include, particularly if you have some personal experience living outside of the U.S.? Are there some international biases you feel also apply in the U.S.? Discuss your list and how you categorized biases with others who have participated in this activity.

A Culture of Competition

In this sorting of people into in-groups and out-groups, a hierarchy is quickly established in dance studios and classrooms. There are those who are a part of the dominant group in dance programs, and those who are not. This orientation to categorize people into dominant and non-dominant classifications is a Social Dominance Orientation (SDO) disposition. Social science research finds a prominent element that supports the culture of SDO is a culture of competition. When dance students are pitted against each other for higher ranking status in the community, there is a corresponding perspective by students that there is an in-group and out-group of students in the learning community. Those that are liked and rewarded, and those who are not liked are not rewarded.[5] Establishing an environment where there is competitive ranking of students heightens the stigma of those who do not rank high in these competitions. For example, when ranking dancers or having a few dancers who are often commended, celebrated, rewarded, etc., dancers in the class receive a signal of what it is and how it is that a student becomes part of the in-group. If the students who are regularly rewarded, for example, are consistently wealthy, White, thin, or carry some other behavioral or visual marker, students equate the privileges to those aspects that connect the in-group members. It also creates clear messages about who is deemed exceptional and who is lacking or deviant from the standards set in a public display for the group. The effects of such a public demarcation of adequacy can have lasting effects on students.

Take, for example, an occurrence in a college course of mine. In the middle of a West African dance class that I was teaching at a college, an African American student began to cry while dancing. After seeing this, at the first opportunity to walk through the classroom as students worked with the movement phrase I provided, I checked in with her. She responded she was fine and did not want to talk about it. This student continued to cry throughout the class while still dancing with full physical investment and commitment to the movement phrases. What initially incited fear in me when I saw her tears—Was there something I did as a teacher that created a negative experience for the student?—after watching over the rest of the class transformed into the feeling that I was witnessing the cathartic experience that movement can engender. The student stayed after class until the rest of the students left and shared with me why she had gotten so emotional. She shared that she was interested in taking dance classes at a local studio when she was a young pre-teen. When she arrived at the dance studio in the new town she had just moved to, the owner explained to her that because she had not been taking ballet, she would need to learn the basics in the classes with the beginners, who were much younger children. Taking those classes was a horrible experience for her. She felt embarrassed and alienated from those her own age. At a time where social interaction with peers was so important, she was placed in a class with children much younger than her, creating a social out-group status amongst her new peers.

For this student, something about taking this class as an undergraduate, non-dance major and being accepted and able to accomplish and enjoy the movement in community with other classmates at her own level of exploration stirred up long-dormant emotion in her about her experiences of not belonging, of feeling like an out-group member in the dance studio of her younger years. She explained that it felt good to be able to dance and enjoy it without feeling like she had to compare where and how she fit in with others around her.

Social dynamics created, maintained, or disrupted in a classroom matter. It matters how an instructor supports every student where they are, while also challenging them to grow on their own terms. It's equally important that this support does not occur in comparison with some sort of rank order with others, or, in the above case, where a student *should* be for their age.

A critical element in the dynamic of competition is the power held by the teacher, who determines the terms, nature, and evaluative measures of how students track their progress or status in the studio or classroom. Without an instructor's relegated leadership and authorization to grade, advance, and promote each student in their progress, the influence of the teacher's perspective would be rather inconsequential or perhaps, only an optional gauge of value or progress. In this way, the importance of power dynamics is a significant factor in establishing and promoting biases, standards, and cultural expectations of the classroom and studio.

Power Differentials and Equity

The power a teacher wields in establishing student rankings is a prominent factor in socializing students to the standards and expectations of the dance field. When biases begin to infiltrate the commitment to include multiple perspectives, they can diminish the ways teachers evaluate different types of dancers and thus affect student rankings in unintended ways. The biases and perspectives of the dominant group, then, become the standard for everyone and every style of dance.

For example, during my college years, an adjudicator's feedback on a modern dance piece I performed illuminated the effects of power coupled with aesthetic preferences. The modern dance piece, choreographed by a guest artist, included livestream video fed from a handheld video camera the choreographer had incorporated into the choreography. This dance work was dense with partnering lifts, catches, and weight-sharing. One adjudicator shared his expectation that there needed to be at least one moment in which dancers balanced on one leg for the work to be an acceptable performance. Because the dance we performed did not have this element, it missed the mark for him. This adjudicator from a classical ballet background had a significant influence in applying his bias for the vocabularies and aesthetics of ballet in the dance competition. While other evaluators from other aesthetic backgrounds and biases felt differently, this evaluator was imbued with the power he shared with other adjudicators to either accept or reject the dance we performed into the top rankings of the competition. In this way, the adjudicator's personal aesthetic preferences were coupled with the power to rank and establish rewards to dancers based on his personal aesthetic preferences.

At events such as this, where there is a panel of experts or adjudicators, I now regularly encourage students to research a bit about the experts judging their work. What type of dance experiences do they have? What type of institutions or companies or creative endeavors have they worked with? This can provide a clearer sense of how the adjudicator understands or sees each work and whether the student aligns with or values that particular sensibility. Encouraging students to consider how their own perspective aligns or does not align with an adjudicator's sensibilities helps students attune to choosing how much value they will imbue to each adjudicator's perspective. This way of adding complexity in student perspectives or decentering a competitive, hierarchical, ranked approach has a number of potential benefits for students. First, it develops a practice for students wherein they do their own research in the field, getting to know various dancers, companies, and educational programs. Second, it helps students learn to place themselves and their own perspectives within the broader field of dance. If there is a particular adjudicator that a student relates to or is intrigued by, this may be a person the student would be encouraged to follow-up with after the dance event. Lastly, asking students to do these kinds of evaluations can stretch the assumed boundaries of the field. There may be an adjudicator that a student has assumptions about. A student may assume the adjudicator or panelist won't be able to understand their work at all, yet receive very valuable perspectives from the adjudicator. Adjudicators may also have moments where their ideas are challenged and they are invited to be more expansive in their evaluation of a form they may not be familiar with. This can be a powerful example for the student of how growth and life-long learning can happen in the field.

These issues of inequity, underrepresentation, misrepresentation, or disregard when applied to groups of people does not need ill-meaning, cruel people to continue to exist. Many of the people within the system of oppressive interactions and institutions are or can be largely unaware of their complicity in the oppression of others until some event causes the disruption or unveiling of this oppressive system. In the above example, the ballet-based adjudicator may have spent much of his dance career with people who carried a similar value system and thus had no reason to disrupt or challenge his own standards. Essentially, all members of a society or community are subject to some level of collective norms, understandings, and messaging from which members of the collective are unable to escape without intentional interventions. The predominance of the ballet aesthetic in U.S. socialization starts early and is pervasive with little disruption until dancers are exposed to other dance forms or learn about differing aesthetic preferences through dance instruction or formalized dance education curricula.

Take, for example, the idea of gender being thought of as a fluid continuum full of variation, rather than as a binary. Think about the experiences of growing up in the U.S. and what messages many Americans have received about gender from the moment a person is born: from asking whether a newborn is a boy or a girl, to pronouns organizing around two dominant gender options, to toys and movies for children being categorized by two genders. Continuing these normative practices around defining gender does not consider the diversity of messages each family or social unit shares for each person who grew up in the U.S., which depend on religious or spiritual beliefs, cultural beliefs, intergenerational dynamics, and what community groups individuals were involved in. How many grew up with the bias that the *man/boy* always lifts the *woman/girl* in dance partnering lifts because *he* is stronger? This is the fallacy of misrepresentation. Instead of acknowledging the physical diversity of bodies and their capabilities apart from sex or gender, many grew up framing dance lifts as gendered, relying on assigned gender roles around physicality and power. It was not until I participated in Edisa Weeks and Homer Avila's partnering workshop, where Edisa was taller than Homer and, thus, often inverted the gender expectations within the partnering work, that I felt affirmed in questioning why women never lifted men. Even decades after that partnering workshop, I still notice that the standard narrative of men lifting women persists. It still is not uncommon for me to hear that the male lifts the female even in this age of non-binary gender discussions and decades of feminist principles present in U.S. social dynamics.

While a person from a marginalized group carries biases, as everyone does, and can therefore have prejudices against others, marginalized groups are not afforded the power on a large scale to create policies, determine who is included or excluded in social groups or institutions, or enforce these prejudices in ways that are socially pervasive. They may be imbued with such power conditionally as a person who maintains the system's values, but these agents often have diminished permanency in positions of power as social out-group members in society.

This is part of the complexity of *intersectionality*, a term coined by Kimberlé Crenshaw, where various social categories carry varying advantages or stigmas and combine in individuals in complex ways. Consider the following scenario. A BIPOC female-identifying dance educator is bestowed the power of gatekeeper in a dance program. This dance educator has privileges as a person in a role that has input in who is accepted into the dance program and who is not. As a member of historically marginalized social identities, however, the dance educator may have a stigma in the deliberations on who is accepted into the program, because of her historically marginalized status. The BIPOC, female educator's contributions may be disregarded if they do not align with the dominant voices in the room. Another instance that could occur is the educator may have even internalized negative stereotypes that result in being more critical of people from another marginalized identity as a survival tool to demonstrate she belongs in the community. She may be more critical of BIPOC female-identifying disabled artists, for example, modeling the discriminatory behaviors she has observed in her colleagues in order to show she belongs in the dominant status category that others benefit from in the room. Various identity markers carry unequal amounts of power.

Race is a pervasive and powerful marker in the U.S. that has been a significant marker of status through the entire history of the country. Racial bigotry and racial prejudice are certainly attributes that any individual can carry and employ whether they are part of marginalized groups or dominant groups. However, it is only members of the dominant racial group who have privileged access to larger institutional systems such as justice and policy systems, mainstream media, and financial institutions and organizations that support, validate, or comply with their perspectives. As we consider the dynamics of power in dance education systems, it is important to consider the intersections between various markers such as gender, race, body size, and ability and how they operate implicitly in systems and daily interactions in our studios and classrooms.

Our educational institutions, administrators, board members, and educators who manage, enforce, and advise on policy may be diverse, but are still agents of a national system that dictate who has the power. In public school education, power structures include local, state, and federal politicians who fund education and make policies, as well as their voting constituents and financial donors. At privately-owned dance schools, organizations, and studios, the funders, whether they be paying clients or philanthropists, have significant influence over institutional decisions. When a person's biases are reinforced by larger social systems, it creates a collective understanding: assumptions that the majority of people concede to as if the biases or presumptions of the dominant groups hold some universal truth. This transforms biases into false truths that the majority of people of a school or educational institution abide by and apply in the daily interactions and operations of the dance community.

The perspectives of marginalized groups, particularly those that run counter to the dominant group's biases, are dismissed, devalued, diminished, excused away, silenced, or attacked. Therefore, the biases of marginalized groups have little to no actionable power or validity unless voiced or touted by the dominant group. This is why it is crucial to understand the dynamics of power in order to understand implicit biases. What seem to be well-informed or universal "truths" may simply be the result of pervasive messaging by systemic power that upholds the preferences and prejudices of the dominant group. When the message is pervasive or is coming from a source that is largely trusted by the society (i.e., news, media, government, educators, etc.), society has a collective understanding of this message, whether that message is true and accurate or not.

ACTIVITY BOX #8: Assumptions Explorer

Some commonly held assumptions that operate as collective understandings in dance include opinions such as Black people can dance and have natural abilities around rhythm; those in wheelchairs cannot dance or at least lack the ability to develop a fully realized movement technique to be applied in concert performances; in order to be a successful dancer, you must be flexible. Name other collective understandings from your own experiences in dance. What are some examples or evidence that you can find that these understandings are not fact or true in a way that applies to everyone?

All Biases Are Not Created Equal

All biases are not created equal. While the same biases can be held by both marginalized and dominant group members in the field of dance education, those biases held only by marginalized groups are not taken up and integrated into society in the same way as those biases held by the dominant group. Rather, biases held, relayed, and enforced by dominant groups in dance education carry more weight, are more readily integrated into the larger field, and are rarely accepted as a perspective held only by a few. Instead, biases held by dominant members of the society as a macrocosm and dance education as a microcosm are assumed to be comprehensively applicable and accepted as common knowledge across the field of dance.[6] Biases that are held only by marginalized groups in the field do not get the same exposure and indoctrination into the field of dance education as those biases held by dominant groups.

This structural power differential inherent to biases operating in society, that dictate who has the opportunity to bestow privileges, resources, or access to others is essential to understand the effects of implicit bias in dance education. No matter the basis of the bias, if decision-makers favor those they consider to be a part of their social group, this is a bias against out-group members. In dance education, the gatekeeper is the person with the power to grant or deny access to the privileges of the in-group. This includes teachers, supervisors, and administrators. If gatekeepers in dance education grant those benefits based on having some sort of commonality that other members of the dance community do not have, this results in **in-group favoritism**. *In-group favoritism* happens, when either those members of the majority in-group or those granted privileges of the in-group, allocate resources, access, or other privileges to individuals that are like them in some way. A seemingly harmless preference, in-group favoritism nevertheless results in discrimination against dancers that are not like those in power.[7] In-group favoritism can be insidious. A social narrative that exemplifies this situation is a dominant, in-group person's intent to help someone in their community. In this case, the grantor is helping a person close to them—a noble and kind task—instead of focusing on the effective discrimination of those that are not close to them. The focus in the dominant narrative is on the help given to a friend instead of the focus being on depriving those that are not part of the in-group of the person granting the favor. Due to the positive narrative frame, this type of in-group favoritism can go unexamined as an inequitable practice.

To further complicate the social strata of in-group and out-group relations in dance, the more nuanced, local relationships of power inequity intersect with the historically marginalized groupings in the larger society. Beyond the U.S. systemic oppression markers like race and class in the application process, dance educators and gatekeepers can also base a decision about an applicant on in-group or out-group markers of familiarity or lack of familiarity. This results in equally-qualified applicants being denied who meet the standard but do not align with some area of personal familiarity, comfort, or favoritism held by the person making selection decisions. Aspects like speech dialects, what a person is wearing, or other behavioral or visual nuances could negatively affect the decisions made by gatekeepers in dance education. Helping a friend, colleague, or stranger who has some common background connection get into your dance program may seem noble or kind. But each time a person with access to resources affords someone with connections or similarities to them an opportunity, this granting of access is an opportunity another person without the connection but with similar qualifications does not get. "While discriminating against those who are different is considered unethical, helping people close to us is often viewed favorably," argues Banaji, Bazerman and Chugh.[8] We are socialized to think of assisting a friend as harmless or even helpful, but this masks the reality that these interpersonal, spur-of-the-moment situations effectively discriminate against those who do not have favoritism with the grantor of the favor.

The field of dance leadership is a clear example of in-group favoritism. The field of dance is a majority female-identifying profession. The historical marginalization of women in the greater U.S. society, however, means that in positions of leadership, like choreographers, tend to be men. In the 2019–2020 U.S. season, for example, men have a higher percentage of representation as choreographers and, thus, more advantages compared to their general percentages in the field.[9] This means that even if women in a local, insular community operate as an in-group in the social strata of the community, women can still incur out-group status in interactions outside of the community due to the greater socialization messages that historically marginalize women in the U.S. The same can be true for out-group members, like White people studying African diaspora dance forms. In the smaller community of African diaspora dance, they operate as out-group members, while in the greater U.S, they may experience some level of in-group status, unquestioned trust in their expertise, or opportunities from their position of racial dominance. These power dynamics not only affect access and selection processes, but they can also affect the very nature of what a person deems beautiful or preferable, affecting how a person feels about a work of art or, in this case, a dance or dancer based on these in-group and out-group markers.

The Persistence and Malleability of Inequity

The nuance of how power is deployed is not only dependent on how small or insular the community is. It is also dependent on the larger social climate. Inequity must alter and shift itself in order to maintain its influence and persistence. This means that the narratives that sustain oppression and inequity are, likewise, mutable. Take, for example, the racial assignation "White." The racial use of the word "White" or how it operates in society, often referenced as Whiteness, is not limited to a simple definition of having White skin.[10] It can signify skin color or phenotypic traits such as thin lips and narrow noses. This term is also used to describe behaviors and social characteristics, which is how it shows up in phrases like "acting White." It also serves as a status of the cultural norm, standard, or universal expectations of high social rank in the U.S. In this way, to refer to White as a racial term means to refer to a malleable, expansive, and dynamic term that applies in many different ways within many different contexts all of which shift in ways that substantiate racial inequity.

Here's an example from the dance world of how malleable implicit messages of power can be in ways that sustain inequity. In administrative responsibilities of managing and maintaining dance programs for businesses or institutions, there are a number of ways that implicit bias manifests. Selection and promotion processes in PK-12 and higher education are rife with implicit bias.[11] An example I have found rather peculiar in my time in education is a penchant for predominantly White institutions or communities to advocate and actively recruit a person of color who does not meet the requirements of the position. Often the fervor is about a passion and commitment to advocating for BIPOC applicants to ensure they are represented in the organization or community. The personal narrative and sense of self developed around helping under-resourced BIPOC dancers, labeled the "White savior complex"[12] in some circles, is undergirded by the implicit narrative that BIPOC students, applicants, or colleagues as a whole tend to be under-resourced as it relates to their ability to qualify at the same or expected level for the position and must be saved by White people in order to be included. This underlying assumption prohibits gatekeepers who choose and recruit BIPOC applicants from thinking beyond their unconscious lower expectations for BIPOC applicants.

In this example, the intentions of the dance educators may be to proactively recruit and support underrepresented and stigmatized BIPOC applicants. But advocating for BIPOC applicants that do not meet the explicit standards set forth for the position ultimately perpetuates the implicit messages of BIPOC people as under-resourced and unqualified applicants. The implicit assumption in this form of advocacy is that there are no qualified BIPOC people or that they are not an adequate fit for some unspoken reason. This takes well-meaning initiatives on the part of well-meaning educators and illuminates how the seemingly anti-racist initiative further substantiates the narrative of lack or deficit around BIPOC applicants. If BIPOC applicants who apply are not meeting the standards set forth for the position, what might be wiser is to examine structural blocks or biases that prevent BIPOC applicants from meeting the standard or examine the internal narratives and logics behind bringing in underqualified BIPOC applicants instead of qualified BIPOC applicants. There may be an internal bias to fill the role of savior of BIPOC applicants that deters dance educators from bringing in qualified, confident, or even emboldened BIPOC applicants that may disrupt the comfort level of existing power structures in the dance program, studio, or educational institution. Again, this is not a hard-and-fast rule or circumstance. The implicit mechanisms that undergird inequity often ebb and flow, shift, and evade our consciousness in ways that serve to maintain the dictates and structural inequities of U.S. systems of oppression. It is crucial to begin to question and examine in a more critical, deliberate, and consistent way the assumptions that operate under our educational decisions and determinations in the field of dance education.

3

Dance Aesthetics

A Site for Bias

ACTIVITY BOX #9: Your Beautiful Journal Reflection

Do a reflective journal submission reading the following questions one at a time and answering them before proceeding to the next question: Describe what beautiful dancing looks like to you. How do you determine what is beautiful? How did you come to know the markers that signify beauty? More specifically, how did you come to know what dances are of artistic quality and what dances are not? How did you come to know the markers that signified that a dance is of quality? Where did you receive guidance, modeling, experience in articulating the words and defining features of a high-quality dance work? Were there people who had a different opinion than you at that time? If so, how did you come to know that the people who shared with you the elements of a quality dance work were experts to be trusted? How did you discern that this expert should be the authority on what determines quality instead of a different person who may have had a different opinion?

༄༄༄

Many of the answers to the questions in the activity above about how we know and learn what is beautiful or what is artistically of quality relate as much to social class, access to power, and group identity as they do to individual preference for one dance over another. The messages and images that circulate via family members, media outlets, and other trusted figures often establish a standard of beauty and aesthetic preferences for individuals. Philosopher Robin James references the work of Jacques Rancière to establish that aesthetics are one way to maintain systems of privilege and oppression.[1] Aesthetics are the delivery method for cultural messages about the power structures of society. As I discussed in the Introduction, implicit bias is a mechanism that is built from implicit memories. These implicit memories are how social notions of common sense are developed that then deliver messages like ballet and modern dance are *high art*, representative of privilege, while dance forms created in the U.S. like hip hop are categorized as social dance, folk dance, or *low art*, and are associated with communities of people not identified as privileged.[2] Whether there is a personal decision to adhere and conform to the standard or to shirk the conforming standard, personal aesthetic choices are often still based on socially ascribed standards of beauty and a person's connection to or rejection of those standards.

How a person defines beauty may indeed be in the eye of the beholder. What implicit bias research confirms, however, is that the eye of the beholder has been exposed to a lifetime of images, behaviors, and messaging that shape a person's ideas of beauty. Part of the process of establishing a sense of beauty in society involves relaying preferences and values through messages and behaviors that operate as a sort of shared common knowledge or understanding, what Immanuel Kant called *sensus communis*, "common or community sense."[3]

Modern dance and ballet are a significant part of dance curricula requirements in many higher education programs because of a "common understanding" that there is less access to depth and rigor in the study of other dance forms. This perception can be interpreted by students from seeing that upper-level courses in dance forms other than ballet and modern dance are far less common in dance programs across the country. Understanding these forms as "lesser" is founded as much on the collective agreement couched in the class status of dancers who study and perpetuate the dominant forms of dance in dance programs as it is based on the practical reasons people provide, such as the fact that there aren't enough teachers with the required terminal Master of Fine Arts (MFA) degree that specialize in forms outside of modern and ballet to teach these dance forms in higher education institutions.[4] Compounding these issues are factors like the economic status needed to access the dance form and the locations in which the form is performed, commodified, and studied, both of which carry messages about social status and also influence decisions about the inclusion of social dance forms. Discussions about social forms of dance are often based on the frequent repetition of the message from people deemed authorities or experts by dominant group members in society, not necessarily on rigorous, informed evidence that offers alternatives to that perspective. The preferences of those who are bestowed the power to speak with authority about the field of dance are based on how people in the society are socialized and steeped in these social hierarchies to trust one person's opinions or findings over another.

3. Dance Aesthetics

The aesthetic values any person has are related to attitudes towards various aspects of visual representation, the language associated with the art form, and how the viewer self-identifies. What a person finds beautiful is influenced by how individuals perceive themselves in relation to society, as well as in relation to those who share their tastes. James explains, "Believing one's aesthetic preferences do and ought to coincide with the general aesthetic norms of one's culture (i.e., ought to be common sense or *sensus communis*) is a form of privilege."[5] Take, for example, the aesthetic messages about white skin color. Cultural messages about beauty and goodness in the U.S. have historically relied on images of white-skinned or light-skinned people who have phenotypically European traits, i.e., straight hair, light skin color, etc. These interconnected qualities that are socially aligned with the wealthy and privileged, who have access to socioeconomic class mobility, reify these traits as aesthetically pleasing. After all, the access that privileged socioeconomic status affords is often a standard for the society and is upheld as a positive goal for those in marginalized, lower socioeconomic classes to strive to attain. These goals are associated with the *good, right, and moral* (all of which are socially constructed). What society has established as good, right, and moral all have visual and qualitative attributes that signal how they are to be perceived in the context of the society or community. Hence, the study of ballet or modern dance are perceived in dominant U.S. culture as good, right, and moral for those who want to succeed in the field, while those interested in dance categorized as social dance forms or some other non-dominant dance form, are not on a pathway of success in the dominant U.S. culture. This disposition to value and center ballet and modern dance over a number of other dance forms that started here in the U.S. is all relative based on dominant culture systems of hierarchy and power, not unquestionable truths.

Many fields, from philosophy to psychology address the process of social indoctrination. In Menakem's book, *My Grandmother's Hands*, he addresses social indoctrination through a psycho-somatic lens.[6] He describes how the reptilian brain operates on the most basic of precepts, "Is this dangerous or safe?" before the more developed and complex cortex of the brain can analyze the event.[7] It is at this bodily, pre-thinking, reptilian level that aesthetics operate. These are the messages of what trusted authorities that are part of the in-groups of a community articulate to society about how society should feel about wholly subjective experiences if we aspire for the privileged status of those dominant in the U.S. culture. In dance education this is what we as dance educators relay to our students about what aesthetics are preferred and what will lead to their success in the field of dance based on what we know of the systemic structures of the field of dance. Aesthetics, the subjective felt sense of an experience, orients danger and constriction—a felt sense of stress, uncertainty, and discomfort—in the body, and safety and expansion—a felt sense of ease, stability, and comfort—in the body. These aesthetic sensibilities are oriented not solely by our own experiences, but also by interventions of *how* to see or experience an event. There is power in the messaging that White, abled, thin bodies are the standard of beauty in the U.S. and result in an expansive feeling in the body of many U.S. audience members that align with dominant sensibilities of what is beautiful in dance. It relays the social stratum that places these White, abled, thin bodies at the apex of value, goodness, morality, and truth—all ideals the brain tends to associate with safety in the dominant tropes of U.S. socialization. This is the reptilian brain feeling its way through the world before the cortex even has the opportunity to think about the response. Menakem further explains, "Often this knowledge is stored in our bodies as wordless stories about what is safe and what is dangerous."[8] For the reptilian, feeling brain, danger messages do not just register bodily harm, but also threats to what we say, do, think, believe in, care about and yearn for.[9] This response to danger does not have to stem from cognitive or situational circumstances, but can be triggered by the mere thought of perceived danger. The ability to quickly activate a danger or safety response from the feeling brain before the thinking cortex is triggered is why messages embedded in aesthetic values so readily activate implicit biases. It is also why the IAT's mentioned in Chapter 2 are so very effective in determining habitual patterns that are oriented around common implicit biases.[10]

In the field of dance, as in the rest of U.S. society, there is a social stratum that signals an unconscious association of constriction and danger in the body when Black bodies are encountered or seen. When Black bodies are then seen in a dance concert, the reptilian brain can still trigger a constriction in the felt sense that then infiltrates how a person sees and feels about Black bodies in the concert performance space. Because this happens without conscious awareness for the audience members at the dance concert, the audience may just be left feeling the constriction and then explaining that they didn't like the concert and don't have language to explain why. If audience members are more skilled in the language of describing and analyzing dance, they might intertwine this subconscious feeling of constriction with elements of the dance to articulate why those particular elements of the dance were unpleasant.

In either case, the person may be completely unaware that what they are expressing is a subconscious fear or discomfort in viewing a Black body, not an aversion to any actual elements of the choreography or performance itself. The person able to articulate some level of their "supporting evidence" for why they did not enjoy the performance may be unaware that their evidence in this case is simply confirmation bias, gathering only evidence that supports the conclusion you intend to assert and disregarding evidence that runs counter to the assertion. If brought to their attention, the viewer may even deny being affected by this reptilian brain trigger. Such a denial may not be an outright lie, because they are not consciously aware the trigger has taken place. There is also the phenomenon of denial of experiencing this aversion to Black bodies because the current social norms of U.S. society tend to be critical of those who explicitly express such biases.

These felt senses experienced in dance performances of course have a fuller range than like or dislike. Of course, we challenge dance students to be more nuanced in articulating what they feel or think about dances they experience. This nuance does not solve the issues that the negative effects of biases may trigger. But in taking the time to process the experience, there is certainly a greater chance of discovering what may be just under the surface of a felt, aesthetic experience when watching or even embodying dance. This is why challenging students to share what they experience when watching or embodying a dance may be the first step in addressing denial of these bias-triggered feelings.

I Don't Have Bias: "The Refusal to Know"[11]

The denial of bias actually preserves and maintains the bias and its structural social feeders of inequity. DiAngelo, in her book, *White Fragility: Why It's So Hard for White People to Talk About Racism*, discusses the notion of grappling with any urges of denial when confronted with the visual markers of race. She shares how the assertion that a person is "color-blind" is counterproductive to disrupting racism. Applying this concept more broadly, to deny racial bias not only sustains the bias of the individual, but also the social cues that created the bias operating in society. DiAngelo asserts that claiming not to see a person's race denies the reality of racism and how different the experiences of many people of color are from White experiences. Not "seeing" race ultimately protects the individual's perception of themselves and socioculturally maintains the White experience as central. In the context of a non-racial but still visual example, I return back to confirmation bias example of the short dancer from the Introduction. A person of the dominant group making the assertion that there is no bias, between a clearly visible difference in the heights of moving bodies, assumes that each person's experience is or should be similar to that of the dominant individual asserting there is no difference.

In this way, it recenters the experience of the person who doesn't *see* differences in height as the experience others must also have as their standard. Essentially, when people with dominant group status ignore differences, they project the personal experiences of the dominant individual onto others, reifying the experience of the person who doesn't "see height," in this case, as normative. Bias works in much the same way. When implicit biases are not named or considered, the effect they have on an individual's perception and, by extension, on their analysis, are not named or acknowledged. Without naming the biases, addressing them is all but impossible. Asserting a distancing or separation from biases masks rather than eliminates elements of that perception bias. Asserting objective distance often requires the observer to disregard aspects of a person's identity. They refuse to consider how those identity-based aspects of the person may be relevant to how the observer perceives and processes what is happening.

In Charles Mills' chapter in *Race and Epistemologies of Ignorance*,[12] he illuminates how denial or willful ignorance of the obvious works to maintain racial inequities. Stanley Cohen, in his book, *States of Denial: Knowing about Atrocities and Suffering*,[13] calls this the rule of not mentioning atrocities and the meta-rule to deny knowledge of the rule. Claiming not to see differences that may be uncomfortable for the observer to address maintains this rule/meta-rule paradigm of silence that precludes the naming and owning of responsibility in the divisive strategies of alienation, subjugation, and inferiority that occur for marginalized people.

The messages that affirm and support underlying privileges and oppressions in society influence what people think they know to be true. In the *Harvard Business Review* article "How (Un)ethical Are You?," the authors explain the effects of these messages: "Exposed to images that juxtapose black men and violence, portray women as sex objects, imply that the physically disabled are mentally weak and the poor are lazy, even the most consciously unbiased person is bound to make biased associations."[14] Watching a higher percentage of bodies of color associated with world, social, and popular dance forms, for example, is part of the categorization process to mark and relegate these forms to a different status than predominantly White dance forms. Then seeing their common status not as central and required in dance curriculum signals that these marginalized forms lack academic depth and complexity to be studied at the level that modern dance and ballet are studied. Watching more White, nondisabled bodies presented in Western (White) concert dance forms affirms that White, nondisabled bodies belong in Western concert dance and are more equipped, qualified, and entitled to perform in those spaces. If the messages from sources people trust as authorities about dance in the society have consistently asserted that ballet is the foundation of all dance forms, many members of society, within the dance community and beyond, are led to believe this misinformation is true. "Trusted" authorities are key to the systemic oppression enacted by the circulation of this fictitious information. Unquestioned acceptance of assertions from established authorities is instrumental in securing methods that perpetuate these inaccurate "truths." These authorities deemed trustworthy (because they are on the news, because they are famous, because they have been hired as educators, because they have been tapped to speak as experts, because they head a company or organization, etc.) share what *sounds* like consistent, familiar, or sensible information within the already-established norms of the society.

Even if there is an outlier, like Misty Copeland as a Black prima ballerina, for instance, the messages communicated about her include the assumption that it is *unusual* to be Black *and* a ballerina. While on its face, this message may sound redeeming and inspiring, it actually reaffirms that ballerinas are rarely Black and that Misty is an outlier or exception to that rule. This message of exceptionalism may not sound problematic initially, because the implicit biases are already well-established in our memory. Experiences find this datapoint consistent with the message that Black people are rarely ballerinas. They result in discussions similar to the one I had with my mother when she asked if I wanted to audition for the magnet school of the arts in my state. I explained to her in my pre-teen years that I didn't want to attend, because there probably will not be Black students like me there.

This socialization of identity markers not only signals for students whether there will be a sense of belonging as a member of the majority or in-group in a dance community, identity markers also create associations between types of dance forms for dancers in dance education programs. Raquel Monroe's article discusses students who pose the question: "I Don't Want to Do African, What About My Technique?"[15] This question speaks to the disconnect between students who identify their studies in their dance genre as rigorous technique while deeming other forms they do not identify themselves with as an undoing of their studies rather than a contributing to their abilities. How can students effectively embody and integrate the works of dancers practicing kinds of dance that aren't widely privileged in dance education? What are ways that dance students can engage deeply in the works of dance forms they have determined are the realm of dance that is relegated to out-group society members? Can the classically trained ballet dancer deepen their learning in a hip hop class on popping and locking? Furthermore, how will students who perceive themselves to be out-group members of a dance genre or community be able to empathize with their dance instructors in their classes to maximize transfer of corporeal information in the dance studio? If societal messaging has created a social divide between a student and how they perceive their dance instructor or the dance form they are studying, how do dance educators close the empathy gap in order to improve the classroom performance of marginalized students?

For years I watched White students participating in West African dance classes make half-hearted attempts to successfully engage with the movement. This always perplexed me with so much discussion from fellow dance educators about the importance of rigor in terms of focus and full physical investment in organizing the body in Western dance forms and little of the same expectation in the elective dance courses where West African dance commonly lives in the curriculum. In my own West African dance classes, I would have discussions with my students about ideas of insider/outsider sensibilities within the movement. In these discussions, White students would often talk about their inability to attain an understanding or any success at the movement because it was so foreign to them. Yet, dance students of color are regularly expected to organize their bodies within European forms of dance. Watching this play out for decades in my own dance training, I posited long before I had any understanding of implicit bias that there was a cognitive identity block for learning wherein some challenges to organizing the body for specific movements comes from a refusal or implicit inability to identify with the groups of people associated with the dance form, or those teaching the dance form.

Striving for social belonging and in-group status in dance is a powerful draw. Belonging in dance means there is an alignment of physically embodied aesthetics with how a dancer chooses to be in the body and present that body in the world. If a student has determined that the "people" who do a dance form are not "their tribe" and not a part of a culture they have a vested interest in empathizing with and understanding, taking in the physical movement of the dance form is all but impossible. This information also becomes pertinent when asking marginalized students to trust and take on the movement of a "tribe" of dancers that they have no association with, even if this new group is the dominant group in the dance community or in society. Students from historically marginalized cultural backgrounds with a strong sense of self and community may find it difficult aligning with a dominant culture that does not make room for or dismisses their culture. They may be unable to connect these dance forms within their bodies, in the dance studio, and by extension in the gradebook. In this way, empathy and a sense of belonging to the group of dancers in the dance community is a crucial piece of this puzzle.

ACTIVITY BOX #10: But Why?

Find a partner for this activity. Share one like, dislike, or opinion. After sharing this statement, your partner can only respond by asking you, "But why?" You must answer their question with as much detail in addressing the why of each explanation you have provided. Do this for a full three minutes. Then switch roles and repeat this activity serving in the other role for three minutes. After taking turns, discuss with your partner what you both experienced or noticed in this activity.

A Note on Empathy and Perception

At this moment in history, when there is such a lack of empathy for those who are not perceived as aligning with one's own beliefs, I ask the question: What happens when the perceiver of an action in a dance class does not experience empathy for the person they are perceiving? Embodying the movement of people perceived to be cultural outsiders or Others speaks to how implicit bias and confirmation bias manifest in an individual's perception and their capacity for empathy. I attended a dance education workshop wherein a discussion spontaneously developed about how to introduce and facilitate conversations with young children about the difficult issues of human cruelty and social injustice. One strategy proposed in the course of the discussion to reduce potential discomfort or harm for young children was to introduce human cruelty and social injustice through examples of how humans mistreat animals. This, according to several participants, could soften the potential trauma of the subject matter for young children.

I had a visceral reaction to this idea. Having grown up seeking to counter the racial trope of my Black body being compared to that of animals, this idea was profoundly repulsive to me. There is a long history in the U.S. of justifying the treatment of Black people, as well as other people of color, through the myths of racial inferiority, which are often conjured through comparing racialized people to animals.[16] In this debunked scientific theory of biological determinism called eugenics, non–Caucasian racial categories were designated to be closer on the evolutionary ladder to animals.

There are a number of social constructs in operation to name here. The first is in the Biblical traditions that "man" was given "dominion" over animals[17] and then doubling down on this idea in the sciences when evolution separates humans from animals by placing humans at the top of the evolutionary chain. The racial construct of White supremacy is also operational, wherein the White racial phenotype is established as the superior phenotype over all other racial categories according to now-debunked eugenics research.[18] As DiAngelo states, "White supremacy is more than the idea that Whites are superior to people of color; it is the deeper premise that supports this idea—the definition of Whites as the norm or standard for *humans*, and people of color as a deviation from that norm."[19] Within my cultural context growing up, there were insults and insinuations based on these themes that, because of my race, I was more like an animal and, therefore, sub-human. These insults were often couched in some reference to a primate. It is why discussions in African American community circles persist, for example, about why, thus far, Disney's only princess narrative set on the continent of Africa was a story of animals. There has yet to be a traditional princess narrative from the continent with human characters in the franchise thus far.[20] Eberhardt also details implicit bias research studies about the pervasiveness of this association of Black people to apes.[21]

With these social constructs, historical contexts, and lived experiences still operating in U.S. culture, I argue the idea that marginalized and oppressed people be substituted or compared with animals being mistreated actually reifies these older social constructs of inequity, disassociation, and dehumanization instead of freeing students from them or providing some more age-appropriate mechanism to discuss oppression and social injustice. This is an example of how insidious signals creep into studios and classrooms. Had I not been present to share with the group the long historical association of stigmatized people with animals, the group may have implemented this plan and by extension reified the very social injustice messages they intended to disrupt.

Herein lies the disconnect between the implicit biases and explicit perception. The implicit bias of marginalized people being akin to animals is triggered in this case. This happened all while the educator who proposed this solution carries an explicit self-perception of seeing herself as a person who cares about the injustices happening in the world and wanting to effect change. The discussion exposed a cognitive dissonance between how those who suggested this solution perceive themselves and the actual negative effect the solution presented in reifying the implicit bias of associating disenfranchised people with animals. This proposed structure intended to protect children would instead bolster the counter-productive bias of stigmatized people being associated with animals and by extension being less than human. The concern that student empathy for fellow humans of color may result in trauma to young children hearing about human injustices resulted in a proposed solution that, in effect, materialized a very old stereotype involving the association of marginalized people with animals. Once these associations are fully solidified as social norms or invisible biases present within U.S. culture, it is challenging but not impossible to make these biases visible and begin the process of destabilizing the social structure of marginalized people as the Other.

The social psychology research on Social Dominance Theory (SDO), described in Chapter 2, considers how empathetic responses and sentiments in human behavior correspond to a person's belief in an SDO framework.[22] According to this research, empathy is affected by a person's perception of whether the person they are trying to empathize with is part of their social group as it relates to this hierarchical structure of social power or not. Those who perceive themselves and their group to have a relatively higher status than other groups also often lack empathy for those outside of their group. The ways that people classify who is part of the in-group and who is not can be based on factors as banal as preference for a favorite sports team or whether they graduated from the same school, and as impactful as categories of people who are the same race or gender. Social dominance research shows an inverse relationship between empathy and SDO. The more a person adheres to SDO the more they frame human interaction around determining whether a person is part of their group or not. Empathy for those that they don't perceive as being a part of their in-group is reduced at best. At worst, SDO results in schadenfreude, taking pleasure in another person's pain or suffering.[23]

The perceived separation of groups of people results in the dissociation of individuals from groups they do not identify with. This dissociation has significant implications in how we perceive and interpret the world and human movement. On a base level, it affects our empathy for one another. Moore and Yamamoto support these findings when explaining the role mirror neurons play in the empathy of movement, feeling a physical resonance with others as they move.[24] Mirror neurons fire both when a person does an action and observes that action in others. This neural discovery lays the groundwork for a physical empathy that is hard-wired in the brain. As Moore and Yamamoto so eloquently state, "it takes experience, conscious effort, and thoughtful reflection to truly understand the meaning of nonverbal behaviors within their varied cultural and social contexts."[25] This is also what it takes to develop empathy that disrupts societal messages that have signaled a person or group of people are not worthy of empathy. For this reason, empathy development in dance studios and classrooms plays a significant role in student learning, empathetic embodiment of movement of other dancers, and the social fabric of dance learning environments. Dance educators should incorporate practices that develop empathy across cultures and hierarchical social orientations in our studios and classrooms. Empathy aids in creating neural pathways that disrupt social hierarchies and support both cognitive and embodied learning in dance classes.

In their book, Mahazarin R. Banaji and Anthony G. Greenwald speak about research on what occurs in the brains of a person when that person does not empathize or relate to another individual.[26] A distinction worth mentioning between the study described in Banaji and Greenwald's book and those studies done on mirror neurons mentioned in Moore and Yamamoto's book is that the study of mirror neurons examines neurons in the premotor cortex that fire while executing a physical action or observing another person executing that physical action. The study explained in Banaji and Greenwald's book focuses on how neurons in the prefrontal cortex fire when thinking of people we identify with and those we do not. When the test subject thought about a person they identified with, the neurons in the prefrontal cortex fired in the ventral region, the area we engage when thinking of ourselves. The test subject's neurons fired in a different area, the dorsal region, when they thought about a person they did not strongly identify with. In Eberhardt's book,[27] she describes the results of Lasana Harris and Susan Fiske's research[28] on extreme out-group members of society. In these studies, images of homeless people triggered the areas of the brain associated with disgust. There was less activity in the parts of the brain associated with seeing another person. Without an ability to identify with those observed, there is a distinction in how the brain processes information gleaned or perceived about the person being observed. How is our perception of a person relevant to our ability to empathize with that person and thus most accurately embody their movement? The potential manifestations of these sorts of divisive byproducts of implicit bias are numerous in the context of dance education environments, and are taken up in the next chapter.

Activity Box #11: An Empathy Experience

Think of a time where you may have felt different or like an outsider in a dance setting. This could be in a dance studio, at a family event, or performance event. What do you remember about either embodying the movement or seeing others dance? Describe what this experience was like for you. What did you do? Was it an enjoyable experience or did you feel some other emotions or sensations? Were there interactions where you spoke with others during the event? What were those exchanges like? What do you remember about learning the movement or watching the performance? List as many details and sensations or emotions as you can about the experience. If you are comfortable, share with others who have also participated in this activity.

4

Biases and Behaviors

Manifestations of Bias

In this section of the book, I share a number of examples of how these implicit biases show up in dance education settings. When considering the ways that implicit bias shows up in dance education environments, there are a number of factors to consider including the organization, the culture, identity, and goals of the dance program, as well as the needs and talents of the population the program serves. Some of the standard aspects of dance education I will examine in this chapter are auditions and other selection processes, curricula and pedagogy, assessment and advising, administrative policies and protocols, as well as the general culture of and interpersonal interactions within the educational setting. Each of these aspects of dance education need to be examined as they animate the social dynamics of historically contextualized discrimination that result in the oppression of colleagues, students, and other partners with an interest in dance education. This chapter will also explore implicit biases that are more individual, local, and non-systemic. While not central to the institutional nature of dance education, these more local biases can result in negative effects on students as well. These are the biases that may be less pervasive in the larger U.S. culture but are more idiosyncratic, based on unique personal biases rarely carried by others in the community. These biases can still cause lasting harm for students.

There are myriad ways in which the negative effects of implicit biases show up in educational settings, and in dance spaces specifically. My first goal is to examine and illustrate how we observe, assess, evaluate, and/or analyze movement through lived examples. I hope to offer new ways to communicate these sensibilities as dance educators so that we do not perpetuate negative assumptions, misinterpretations, or stereotypes of students, colleagues, and applicants in dance education settings. Misinterpreting, devaluing, or overvaluing people's behaviors and dance performances with no awareness of the educator's personal bias results in personal harm to marginalized members of a community. For all members of the community, it causes missed opportunities for trust, understanding, and connection. These manifestations of bias take the form of behavioral interactions, meaning that my illustrative examples look at what a person or people are doing, saying, or deciding, then generating meaning from that. This can take place in faculty meetings, classroom interactions, and teachers observing students outside of class in social settings.

Biases color the interpretations of physical movement—i.e., how a student dances, what body language is taking place when a person is speaking in a conversation, or how a student sits or stands during class time as a teacher is speaking to the class. Short of video recording movement, the memories, messages, and biases developed through socialization are the organizing systems left to perceive movement after the movement experience has ended. Even then, the historical and social moment a dance is performed in can have an impact on the meaning of that dance. For example, when I was touring a lighthearted, playful, and engaging step dance called "Bushwhackers," choreographed by Kim Tapp, a poignant moment of the importance of context and its influence on interpretation happened. While the dance had no direct relationship or intended commentary about the presidential Bush family, my professor found herself about to introduce this dance in the rotunda of the Texas State Capitol building in the years after George W. Bush had left the position of governor to pursue a presidential run. She grabbed the microphone and with calm, ease, and grace introduced the dance troupe and the university name, avoiding stating the title of the piece in that space. To avoid the misreading of the dance as some nod, insult, or even threat to George W. Bush, the professor made a spontaneous choice not to state the name, "Bushwhackers," in the Texas State Capitol building.

Had she said the name in that charged political space, the erroneous connection of the title of the dance to the former governor could have infiltrated how audience members interpreted the dance, the dancers, or even the dance program. The space and historical moment the dance was being performed in had a meaningful influence on the dance because of the way its title could be perceived to be commentary about the Bush family. Of course, those performing the dance who opposed Bush's political leanings were also affected in this performance context. The dance was now inscribed with a secret, irreverent double meaning that offered up an opportunity to embody protest to the political leanings of G.W. Bush. The enthusiasm of those loving this covert message infused a more enthusiastic engagement in performing the dance. This dynamic of the dance would not exist for audiences or performers outside of this specific location and historical moment. The potential of a perceived connection to G.W. Bush was not made before this performance, and did not linger after. The interpretation of a video recording of this performance with no information about the setting or performance date would not invoke the same possible meaning or association to G.W. Bush. The variation of interpretation increases when dances are performed live, because when dances are performed live, there is never an exact repeat of that single performance or performance context. Each live embodiment of the dance is different even in the most minute detail variation and in the historical moment of the performance.

So, what of memory, the place the live dance performance arrives after the lived experience of the movement has ended? Examples of how bias operates in remembering the details of an event have been a significant area of study in the judicial system. Levinson considers how memory is constructed through the implicit biases of jurors using two phenomena: (1) misremembering, or memories that contain inaccurate details, and (2) forgotten information, or memories where pertinent details are redacted by the mind. These glitches of the mind are not random, but when collected and tracked, illuminate the biases of the juror-observer.[1] Portions of the juror's memories that were consistent with their own bias remained intact while elements that did not align with stereotypical attributes of individual people tended to either get revised in the memory, recalled with details that aligned with the bias, or tended to be lost to the juror's memory altogether. Levinson found there was a higher prevalence of misremembering that was linked to bias as opposed to simply forgetting information. Also, the more factors the brain has to process in the task at hand, the higher the chance for errors in judgment. While this concept is taken up more thoroughly in Chapter 5 in my discussion of a concept called "**cognitive busyness**," it is worth mentioning here as a factor that increases the frequency of false memories. This busyness includes how complex the details are that need to be remembered, as well as the level of stress and the level of distraction involved in recalling a memory. For those who have ever taken a dance class or been charged with distilling the physical experience of movement into a finite, language-based notation or evaluation record, this list of details, stress, and distraction affects the accuracy of memory and, therefore, can leave the educator susceptible to implicit biases influencing the analysis or assessment of dance students. In dance education, these studies lead me to wonder how, in a classroom or dance studio, are implicit biases rescripting what actually took place in live exchanges, from class discussions to across-the-floor combinations? What details of an exchange or performance are subverted or discarded because it does not fit into the preconceived notions we have about a student or colleague?

I had a thought-provoking conversation with graduate students about how to respond to students when the body language of the student at rest during lectures is perceived as disrespectful by the teacher. This conversation came up in a graduate-level movement observation class where students were being challenged to both name how they interpreted what they saw in their classes and then how they *know what they know* about how they interpret student behavior in class. In this conversation, I shared examples of moments in which I erroneously thought that a quiet student was either disinterested or disengaged because they were lying on the floor as they listened to class discussion in a dance studio. In dance, as we observe human movement to glean impressions, narratives, nuance, and artistic or technical execution, I suggested that graduate students address what they are seeing and how they would rather the student exhibit their attention in class as a way to make explicit what their personal biases are, and by extension, communicate what their expectation for engagement looks like in the class. This curiosity and critical self-reflection about how we perceive movement should take place not just during moments of observation but also during moments of embodying movement.

In the process of transitioning from the experience of movement (visual or physical) through the filter of socialization into memory construction, unconscious biases serve as an instantaneous editor that removes details inconsistent with our unconscious beliefs and reforms other details in a way that supports those unconscious beliefs. The moment movement has passed from the present, construction of memory begins. Memory is just as much socially constructed by the cultural background of the observer and the influence of trusted opinions, as it is constructed by what is taking place and what is in the environment in the moment of performance. The mover/observer may also be primed by unnoticed elements present in the room that are not the subject of the class. So, the movement itself, the bodies doing the movement, and any other sensory information taken in during the class can also affect the interpretation.

At times, the dance students and dance educators' interpretations of experiences align as members of a similar cultural background. In other instances, the dance students or dance educator's background may vary from each other or even from the social norms in place in society. In the above experience I had performing "Bushwhackers" in college, I had experiences growing up in a cultural environment where I regularly saw step dances being performed and also performed in step dances. This afforded me a closer orientation and understanding of the aesthetics of step dance even though my dance colleagues and professor did not have a similar cultural exposure to the dance form. My social norms growing up enthralled with ballets like The Nutcracker also included regular trips to African American cultural events, historically Black colleges and universities in the area, and Black performers presenting work in my area. For a time, I was the only Black dancer performing in "Bushwhackers." The professor who cast me in the work did so intentionally, with an understanding that I had a social and historical connection to the aesthetics of the dance form. I was able to provide feedback about accuracy, nuance, and style both through movement demonstration and verbal feedback from my cultural connections and experiences with the dance form. But how does this affinity and attention to observational accuracy happen?

Moore and Yamamoto propose solutions for more accuracy in observation and analysis. This conversation is applicable in dance education settings for instructors and students. It is applicable for instructors who provide movement experiences, observe student engagement with or performance of the movement, and analyze that engagement or performance for the purposes of student development and assessment. This discussion is also valuable for understanding student observation and analysis within the classroom setting. It also provides a context to more fully understand how a student attunes their analytical sensibilities based on what the teacher models about how to see, talk about, and embody movement.

Moore and Yamamoto articulate the factors that result in deviation between what movers intend and what observers interpret. The authors explain:

> The extent of divergence is dictated by myriad factors: the clarity with which the mover conveys his or her intentions, the acuity of the observer's perception, the similarity of cultural and social backgrounds between mover and observer, their personal familiarity to each other, as well as their motivations and needs to understand one another. The clearer the movement expression, the more acute the observer, the more similar the backgrounds, the greater the personal familiarity, and the stronger the urge to understand, then the greater the congruence is likely to be between the mover's intentions and the observer's interpretation. [...] if the movement expression is ambiguous (or if the mover purposefully attempts to disguise her or his intentions), if the observer is inattentive or inexact, if the two individuals come from dissimilar backgrounds, if they are also strangers to one another, and if they do not need or want to understand each other, then we may assume that the divergence in their perspectives will be great indeed.[2]

When considering these factors of divergence between how the observer and mover perceive movement in the context of implicit social attitudes, these factors of divergence become problematic. Socialization and training experience is what helps both the mover and observer understand exactly what the terms, frame, implied rules, and aesthetics are of the movement context they are in. The term *clarity*, for example, is dependent upon what the genre and culture of the movement is that is being performed. In the classroom, it may also be dependent on what the learning objective, rubric, or focus of the day is as set by the instructor. Spatial clarity, for example, may appear to be ambiguous if the observer is unaware of what the spatial reference of the dance form is. If the dancers are orienting toward cardinal directions—to the sun, the moon, or a particular figure in the performance space, for example—the observer that is accustomed to orienting toward physical building structures or stage directions may perceive the spatial orientation to be ever-shifting and ambiguous.

When the authority to observe and evaluate dance performance is based on the viewer's personal familiarity with or similar background to the mover, this raises questions of equity and access. While I do acknowledge the importance of understanding the aesthetic, cultural, and power dynamics of a movement context in order to accurately assess and interpret movement, there is a way in which in-group members of the field of dance education reify what is asserted by the dominant group members in the dance education field, as opposed to the sensibilities of marginalized dance forms or dance groups. With no consideration, questioning, or critical analysis of a marginalized group within the field of dance education, there may be missed details or aspects that go unconsidered in perceiving what is present in the movement. There may be valuable aspects that go unexamined when the majority of people in the group, particularly those with more power and privilege in the room, are evaluating a performance from similar perspectives, backgrounds, and training. This groupthink, coupled with the privileged status of the viewer's perspective, reinforce the voices of those majority and dominant figures in the movement observation event, shrinking space for others to share alternative or expansive ways to perceive and analyze the movement.

Manifestations of bias can be gleaned and evidenced by statistical data like that provided by NASD I shared in the Introduction that tracks a number of different trends in hiring practices and student enrollment for affiliated dance programs. Through asking the right set of quantitative questions to collect the relevant datasets, biases can become evident. Questions could include: What are the percentages of BIPOC students in our program, and how do our numbers compare to the national percentages of BIPOC people in the U.S.? If I as a dance educator track the grades I provide in courses by race or gender, do I disproportionately give higher grades to a particular gender or race of student? When our program posts job announcements, when, how and in what proportion are historically marginalized groups—i.e., BIPOC, LGBTQ,[3] disabled, etc.—applying to those jobs? What is the racial breakdown of students who are selected to receive awards in our dance program? Do they mirror the demographic percentages of the student population? These datasets can indicate what is occurring in the educational setting that otherwise may not be evident to the whole community. This data can be collected from a number of different procedures and protocols in education. It can be collected in demographic record-keeping of the hiring pool and hiring selections, student pool including who is accepted and who is offered funding, and in grading as organized by demographic categories in classes, in the program, or in different types of classes (i.e., theory and writing courses, or choreographic process course, studio technique courses, non-major or major courses). Data can also be collected from other notable selection processes in educational programs such as excellence awards or other honors bestowed on students and employees. What are the demographics of the educators who are considered for and/or granted awards or promotions? For example, looking at demographic data can illuminate the effects of bias in selection processes, gatekeeping measures, and any quantitative deviation from the demographic ratios of people from which selections are made. For example, if a dance program has a demographic percentage of 75 percent White students and 20 percent Black students, while the demographic pool of applicants to the program is 40 percent White students and 30 percent Black students, implicit biases may very well be operating in the dynamics of the dance program.

Keeping track of datasets in a dance program like those mentioned in the previous paragraph and in the NASD data from the Introduction can pinpoint the effects of implicit bias in a number of different areas that may otherwise go unnoticed or unfounded. Tracking the demographic breakdown of grades students receive can illuminate potential bias in how a teacher is assessing students, or even how effectively that teacher is communicating class performance expectations and content. The data gathered about the percentages of underrepresented or historically marginalized populations in search and selection processes can also illuminate potential issues in rubrics used to evaluate applicants, or the problematic logics in the deliberation process that serve to maintain the negative effects of bias.

Problematic or inconsistently applied logics can then become apparent as double standards, undefined or unstated criteria or standards being used to deliberate, or moveable logics—stated reasoning that applies only to some but not to all who are being evaluated or reviewed. Setting clear and explicit criteria that applies to each candidate under review helps to suppress any unconscious effects of biases. Of course, I have certainly been in situations, particularly early in my teaching career, where it is clear and evident that the set of criteria or rubric that I have developed is not effective. This has happened in at least two ways. One is that there is a very specific student issue that calls for a different or amended approach to evaluation: an injury, for example, that allows a student to keep dancing but with modifications. The second circumstance is that there is a significant factor of student performance I did not anticipate that needs to be explicitly addressed but is not accounted for in the rubric or criteria designed before the class began. In both of these cases, it is important to either make the adaptation clear and explicit to the entire pool of students, or wait until the next cycle of the process during the next term to apply it. When you have an outlier in the pool of applicants that seems to warrant an exception to the criteria, the criteria might be inadequate or in need of revision. The criteria do not consider in an inclusive and equitable manner the pool of students being reviewed if there is one or more in the pool that seem not to fit the criteria in some way.

For another example of this double-standard phenomena, I will share a personal example of a body weight bias in the use of physio-balls in a workshop I attended. The participants were provided physio-balls for some of the activities and for their own personal comfort or physical needs during the long meeting days. The facilitators requested at the start of the workshop that participants not sit on the balls to avoid any balls from bursting. But as the days wore on, some participants did casually begin to sit on the balls during lecture sessions. When I observed this and attempted to do the same, I was singled out and asked not to sit on the balls. I was the only participant asked to adhere to the request after the initial announcement about not sitting on the physio-balls, even though a number of students ended up sitting on the balls.

As both the one fuller bodied and only Black participant, coupled with the socialization context of a fuller bodied Black woman's lifetime of messages received from the dominant culture, I knew there were a number of implicit biases that undergirded the inconsistent enforcement of this rule. Thicker bodied people are suspected to be lazy or unhealthy coupled with the historical cultural messaging that Black people are lazy, which undergirds much of dominant culture throughout the history of the U.S. There is the history of the expectation that White bodies should be or are responsible for policing and surveilling Black bodies to help them attune and assimilate to dominant culture expectations that also resonates in this example. Yet another factor of dominant culture existing in the room is of White innocence, where White students are seen as more innocent than students of color, and a racial epistemic ignorance, a performance of *not knowing* that the inequity is taking place.[4] These are some of the silent messages already present in this situation that a marginalized student is often hyper-aware of from their own lived experiences, whether from messages about weight, skin color, or being the only member of your identity in a room. These messages are all reinforced for me as a fuller-bodied

Black woman whether the thinner White participants or instructors in the room are conscious of it or not. These messages are rescripted the moment the instructor asks the only Black, full-bodied participant in the room to adjust without asking the same of the other participants.

This outlier or exception in how classroom criteria are applied may also take place when those being reviewed are in some way part of an in-group that accounts for a positive bias in support of the applicant even though the criteria have not been met. This in-group or favored status of a person is another manifestation of the negative effects of bias. When there is some personal and positive connection between the person being reviewed and those deliberating, the opportunity for bias to affect the deliberation and evaluative processes is high. While seemingly harmless, helpful, and kind, the common narrative of heart-warming storylines in the news cycle, enacting a personal favor of providing assistance, or greater positive consideration because of a close personal relationship or familiarity is still a manifestation of bias. What is left out of this seemingly innocuous help is what is not being equitably provided for others. What often affords a person favoritism in these circumstances are structural and unstated familiarities and affinities such as race, class, profession, gender, etc. Without extending the same considerations and support to the others being reviewed, this is an inequitable practice, however well-intentioned the initial urge to help.

Assigning permanent character assessments or attributes to students in a way that results in treating a student differently than the rest of the class is a potential site for bias to manifest. For example, if there is a student that has not had any previous experiences of being late, missing deadlines, or having other issues that may negatively impact their class performance, excusing the student from the established consequences of these infractions reifies a dominant narrative that teachers have favorites in a class that do not receive the same consequences for infractions as other students do. If this character valuation continues to be used to excuse the student from equitable enforcement of rules, expectations, or rubrics, the dance educator is exhibiting a bias in favor of the student.

Two things are problematic here. One is that there is an assumption that character or even a collection of behaviors is fixed and does not change for students. Another issue is that this fixed character assessment (in the mind of the instructor) is used to modify or amend explicit guidelines, protocols, or assessments. This pattern of behavior exhibited by educators or committees assessing student performance and evaluating student infractions reinforces that there is no fair and equitable treatment of students, and that some students bear the brunt of consequences because they are seen as "bad" in the eyes of those determining their character.

This can also be detrimental to the "good student" in the class. If the student characterized as "good" begins to have challenges or begins to deviate from previous performance in class, this may be due to a major life event that needs addressing. Disregarding those changes observed in class then results in a lag in addressing what may be a significant change in that student's life for which they may need support. Catching these behavioral shifts in class performance early are beneficial for identifying and addressing challenges that may not be apparent inside the classroom such as family crises, health issues, socioeconomic challenges or other changes in availability of basic needs for that student. It also calls educators to challenge implicit biases that may keep some students under constant surveillance in anticipation of less-than-stellar behavior, while leaving other students immune or invisible to this surveillance, even when those students may also be struggling.

After reviewing any statistical data collected around potential inequities in your dance schools and programs, take a moment to breathe. It is important to remember the practice of noticing, sitting in, and attending to any cognitive dissonance that may arise in moments where the data or other indicators point in a different direction than the commonplace beliefs or personal perceptions about the field of dance, dance education, or your program. Taking time for internal reflection may result in realizations that what the data illuminates about your teaching, your program, or even about the field of dance education may feel different from how you personally perceive the field. Perceptions that may have been well-intentioned yet mistakenly perceived to be true are simply opinions or felt senses of the state of equitable practices in the dance education field. What happens when you track your thoughts and internal dialogue as you sort through how you feel about this data, your role in the field of dance education, and your approaches thus far to the state of equity in the field of dance education. Focus on noticing your thoughts, emotions, and physical sensations without judging them as you notice them. Track them with curiosity of what arises letting go of any urges to push whatever arises away or reject it. Hold it in your awareness with full consciousness of its presence without attempts to fix, celebrate, or judge whatever arises. The urge to suppress or attach to what arises is what further solidifies the way the mind asserts its sense of itself and its established bias. Suppressing our reactions prevents the aspects of unconscious bias from moving into conscious awareness, where they can be addressed, examined, and transformed should the personal goal be to move beyond the implicit bias.[5] When ready to move on into a different way to frame and organize the categories of how implicit bias manifests in dance education, proceed to the next section.

ACTIVITY BOX #12: Body Scanning When Bias Wells Up

Think of a moment of discomfort around a misunderstanding, wrong assumption, microaggression, or stereotype triggered by a bias you have. Once you have thought about an episode, close your eyes and return to that moment. Think about as many details about the event as possible. As you return to this moment, track any sensations or thoughts that come up in your brain-body. Consider noticing your heart rate, your breathing, your joints or muscles. Maybe you feel warmth, cool, or some other unique sensation in a certain area in your body. Can you remember any sensations connected to words you said or heard others say in the exchange? Take some time to journal about this event with a particular focus on tracking and describing what you noticed in the way of sensations in the body. Consider doing this practice soon after these events occur to track your sensations in a way that helps note when the discomfort takes place and how it manifests.

Implicit Bias in Mind, Word, and Deed

Implicit biases show up in mind, word, and deed: in the internal perspectives a person thinks, what a person says verbally, and in behaviors the person enacts. In the category of mindset or what social scientists may term disposition, there are assumptions about people, expectations of others and what they may be thinking, what they may do, or what you expect their underlying motivation to be in their thoughts or behaviors. Those attitudes and dispositions in the mind then influence language and how we organize ideas verbally. These dispositions also affect behaviors and the decisions of what actions to take in various contexts.

Now I ask you to stop for a moment and take a breath. Notice the categorization of this information shared in the paragraph above. It is organized in a way that separates mind from body, thinking from doing, rather than considering the integrated and interrelated nature of how these elements sit inside a person as a whole. The practice of bringing this sort of habitual noticing into daily practice is a valuable exercise in repatterning the negative effects of biases in daily life. Take a moment to think about other ways you might restructure this list of manifestations of implicit bias.

As you read further about each manifestation of implicit bias, consider new ways of categorizing and organizing these ideas. Maybe there is a way to organize them by where they tend to occur in your daily life, or you might consider what role you may be playing most often when they occur. I ask you to consider this because, while I move forward with this triad of ways to think about bias, it is important to know that there are other ways, angles, and perspectives to consider in how they may show up in your personal life and in educational settings.

This categorization method is also another wonderful example of how socialization colors organizational categories we have at our disposal. The separation between mind and body that René Descartes proposed has become such a significant conceptual frame in the Western world, so much so that the notion of organizing a phenomenon by its internal mental manifestations and its external behavioral aspects may seem banal for some. In our smaller microcosm in the field of dance education, and even more so the smaller group of somatic movement specialists working in dance education who believe in the integration of mind and body, this divide may throw up a red flare for how problematic separating the mind from the body can be.[6] I acknowledge that, but carry forward the perspectives of researchers in the field of implicit bias research for us to examine through our own lenses of embodied learning, where mind and body are often considered as wholly integrated and not separate at all.

Mindset Matters

Students' assumptions and expectations based on previously established social messages that develop into implicit memories that then enforce stereotypes can be a manifestation site for implicit biases in our dance classes. Assuming or expecting students to behave a certain way based on how the educator has misinterpreted social cues or markers of identity can show evidence of prejudices applied in the classroom. These prejudged behaviors may stem from sociocultural stereotypes commonly found in the U.S., how the student was perceived in previous classes with the instructor, or how relatives of the student may have been perceived in previous classes. This is a human tendency to assume that one type of person will fill a certain role because the implicit memories have organized experiences in a clearly recorded pattern of what type of social markers fill specific roles.

It is exhibited in the moment we ask only the Asian-appearing student if they would be interested in learning an Asian dance form instead of the modern dance form the majority of their classmates are taking. Then it turns out that Asian-appearing student grew up in Mexico and feels no particular connection to or interest in Asian culture. The teacher has erroneously assumed based on visual markers that the student would be interested in Asian dance forms. A teacher's implicit memories are also in operation when a teacher assumes the late assignment yet to be submitted is from a student who struggled with staying on task and submitting work on time the year before not realizing the student did a tremendous amount of maturing and improving since the last class and submitted early. This assumption is based on implicit memories and assumptions that a student's character and disposition in class is permanent. I even once had a professor in an individual meeting begin to plot ways I could work a job outside of school at local bars to afford school, when I had no need for additional financial support in school. I was perplexed about the source of her assumption. My fellow Black student colleagues explained she offers that to all the Black students who arrange meetings with her. This professor assumed that all the Black students in her classes were in economic need of extra work based on the social messages about pervasive Black socioeconomic disparities in the U.S.

Another form of mindset bias that shows up in dance education is **cultural cloning**, a tendency to a "systemic reproduction of sameness."[7] Essed and Goldberg's definition of this term applies seamlessly to the systemic replication of White homogeneity in high-ranking positions in dance education. This speaks to a pattern of repeatedly placing the same type of person in a position based on their gender, race, or ethnicity. For example, if a program director has only been exposed to artistic directors who are White males, the program director may only consider White males as the most appropriate type of person to fill the role of artistic director. The human brain unconsciously tends to think of the most appropriate prospective type of person to fill a role. This can include a person looking like and having similar identity markers as the majority of the people who have previously filled the role.

An example of this cultural cloning is evident in the Dance Data Project.[8] In the 2019–2020 Season Overview study of the top 50 U.S. dance companies, 72 percent of the works shown in the 2019–2020 season were choreographed by men, even though in 2019 women made up 71 percent of the dance field.[9] While women make up a majority of the field of dance, men are still filling higher ranking or more exclusive positions in the field. In terms of cultural cloning, the high incidence of males attaining leadership roles in the field is indicative of replicating the historical bias that men should be in leading, exclusive roles in society.

The tendency to replicate our sensibility of what type of person should fill a particular role could also manifest in the type of students or student body a dance program has previously accepted. A lack of openness to considering a student who may not look like or present as a similar type of student the program has had in the past can affect whether or not the program considers accepting a new *type* of student. If the preference in the human mind is to replicate sameness on the terms established by our socialization (i.e., gender, race, class, able-bodiedness, etc.), it is important to identify this mental habit in the selection processes of a program in order to prevent dismissing a wholly qualified student that varies from the precedent in gender, race, ethnicity, class, or even age and other formulaic considerations.

Another manifestation of implicit biases in mindset comes in the way of what Levinson calls misremembering, which I previously mentioned in the Introduction.[10] In brief, *misremembering* happens when the mind deletes memories that do not align with implicit biases already existing in the mind, or alters memories in a way that supports the existing implicit beliefs and implicit memories experienced. Levinson was able to track the connection between inaccurate memories of what jurors remembered about testimony provided in court to a pattern of common stereotypes or structural social biases consistent with the messages received in dominant culture socialization. Levinson accomplished this using the documentation of testimony given to compare what was actually said during testimony to what jurors remembered during deliberations. If you think of the ephemeral nature of dance, it is not difficult to see the potential influence and harm the unconscious effects of misremembering could have in the dance studio or classroom. Without some mechanism of objective record-keeping, documentation, or an outsider's perspective, there is no way for an educator to become aware of this unconscious pattern of the mind as it aggregates memories within existing subconscious social frameworks. How, as educators, are we to determine whether the marginalized student who just executed a phrase across the floor was not exhibiting their full physical effort or whether the educator's mind simply aggregated the information received based on what memories and assumptions about the student were already there? There is also no way, with simple observation and no daily record-keeping, to track the frequency of when a student was or wasn't meeting expectations in studio work over the length of the academic term. The mind could also aggregate the number of instances of student performance over time in a way that negatively affects and does not accurately represent student performance.

It is challenging to detect the inconspicuous cognitive processing of any individual and even more challenging to determine the role of unconscious effects of dominant culture socialization in any circumstance. This is why the tedious, specific, and quantitative work of social cognition research on implicit bias has been so very powerful in tracking the effects of socialization. To understand and track these mental processes, it is incumbent on those who are committed to disrupting its negative effects to learn about how dominant culture messages have affected our ability to be equitable.

Language Matters

The influence of biases in mindset quickly shows itself in negative effects evident in language. Bias can result in microaggressions, stereotypes, and character assignations that are based less on behavior than they are on identity. These biases can become evident via what a person says. Even if the language on its face is complimentary, the message behind the words may still reify assumptions about a person that are bias-based.

An example of how stereotypes manifest in language in dance is conferring on a Black dancer a natural talent for physicality or rhythmic coordination while asserting that White people don't have this natural dance ability. While this may seem complimentary, the socialization of stereotypic assignations of physical prowess and natural effortless physical talent to Black bodies, while White bodies are associated with intellect and rigorous training, results in biased assumptions that White dance work is more rigorous, intellectually stimulating, and worthy of study, funding, etc. It can manifest when Black dancers, whose creative work involves as much study and preparation as White dancers, is relegated to unexamined entertainment with no attention to the creative rigor and artistic nuance of the work. In this case, Black bodies are afforded less credit or merit and, instead, are assumed to have had to work less to develop the resulting performance. Jesse Phillips-Fein and I articulate an example of this in the following passage:

> It is through the construct of Whiteness that dancing "naturally" is seen as an activity that belongs on Black bodies, while simultaneously relegating these bodies and their dances outside the realm of "acceptable" and "proper" dancing. In this configuration, not only are Others more likely to be overrepresented by their corporeality, their perceived physical skills are seen to be the result of innate ability, not acquired skill. This further devalues the expertise of Black dancers, seen not as the result of hard work and training but rather as an expression of "natural embodiment" assigned to Black bodies.[11]

In any circumstance that a person is not thought of as an individual, but, rather, as a part of a culture and all of the identity politics, behaviors, traditions, and cultural artifacts that are ascribed to that culture, there is a high potential for often unintended manifestations of bias to occur. A participant in a workshop session I was leading asked the great question about acknowledging a person's culture without reifying stereotypes. She asked whether treating people as individuals and not as carriers of the whole of a culture means we are unable to compliment a person on aspects of their culture, such as garb, food, etc. The trepidation comes when a person assumes an individual's connection to a culture based on some visual marker, rather than on what a person has already shared about their connection to a cultural identity. I personally, for example, feel myself reserve my excitement or curiosity about commenting about a person's culture until an individual takes the lead sharing whatever it is they are comfortable sharing about their own culture and connection to that culture. For me to take the lead in assuming any particular narrative I have envisioned about a person's connection to a particular culture invites the potential for misunderstandings and erroneous assumptions. In systems of oppression in the U.S., those in the dominant culture are more often perceived as individuals with unique interests, traditions, artifacts, or behaviors, with varied backgrounds while those ascribed to be of a non-dominant culture are seen through a broad lens of the cultural factors people know about that culture.[12]

In the verbal manifestation of bias, a large carrier of bias comes in the form of **microaggressions**.[13] *Microaggressions* is a term created by Chester M. Pierce in 1970 describing "brief and commonplace daily verbal, behavioral, or environmental indignities, whether intentional or unintentional, that communicate hostile, derogatory, or negative racial slights and insults toward people of color."[14] Some examples of microaggressions are asking people of color where they are from; repeatedly mispronouncing the names of people of color or calling them by another person of color's name; and giving compliments about a student's performance that explicitly key in on their race as a contributing factor for giving the compliment. Underneath these verbal insults are a range of racially-charged assumptions and expectations.

Asking a person of color where they are from assumes that, as a person of color, they must not be from the U.S. Ironically, White people are also not indigenous to the lands on which the U.S. sits. The dominant culture's messaging, however, has socialized people not just in the U.S. but abroad as well to believe that the U.S. is the land dominated by, and nation originating with, White people.

Repeatedly mispronouncing names communicates that the individual whose name is being mispronounced is an outsider or foreigner, and that there will be no intention to honor the family who named them or the culture their name comes from. Even in a seeming compliment, if the person being complimented is explicitly noted as a person from a group that is not usually complimented on the specified aspect, the person giving the compliment is relaying it in the context of assuming many would not expect the person to be successful at the highlighted feature. Take, for example, complimenting a Ghanaian student on how articulate they are in their pointe work. This compliment comes with the assumption that the student was not expected to be as articulate as they are and reinforces the stereotype that Ghanaian students are usually not as articulate in dancing en pointe as this particular student.

Euphemisms are another way that biases show up in speech, particularly when assessing the character of a person. These are words or phrases that soften the delivery of offensive, harsh, or prejudiced messages. In this way, they serve to communicate harmful, insensitive, or racist ideas packaged in socially acceptable language. An example of this I found in my years of evaluating student infractions while teaching in PK-12 schools is the phrase "But [insert student's name] is a good kid." When this phrase is deployed while discussing student infractions or determining consequences for poor behavior or student performance, it usually signals those students established as *good* students do not warrant consequences. I, too, often found that articulating that a student was good was a way to excuse them from receiving consequences for their actions.

I kept wondering what my colleagues thought happened to good students who regularly received little to no consequences for actions they saw others receive harsher consequences for. In my mind, this develops entitlement, superiority, and hubris that sends the message to the student that they are unconditionally above reproach and privileged, because they have been identified in the social strata of the school as "good." We might also question exactly what a person means by *good*. There are implicit values not being unpacked if there is no clear rubric or determination that explicitly articulates the values ascribed to *good* students.

Behavior Matters

This brings us to the final category of how biases show up: in behaviors. I return to the example described before about the physio-ball directive that was only enforced for me, the one Black, curvy participant. The behavior of only asking the one Black participant to get off of the physio-balls is an example of what I call a movable logic, and points to the issue of double standards. Treating one student differently than others based on your personal assessment of how you perceive their behavior is a manifestation of bias. No matter an educator's personal feelings or even interpretations about a student's intent, it is important for educators to apply any explicit rules, protocols, or expectations equitably across all students.

Here it is important to distinguish the difference between "equal" and "equitable." Equal would be to treat each student exactly the same, no matter their needs. An example of equality would be requiring every student to take an English as a Second Language course no matter their proficiency in the English language. To be equitable, an educator would provide what is needed for each student's success on an individual basis. Creating an equitable classroom may mean different things for different students. What should remain constant, however, is the expectation of growth and any explicit factors a teacher articulates as a model for student success. In this way, an educator can both meet the student where they are while still investing the necessary encouragement, support, and challenge needed for student growth and successes. Often, showing favor or contempt by way of behavior in a classroom or studio can hinder student success. For those favored, this favor signals they do not have to work as hard to be successful, and for those stigmatized, this stigma signals being successful in the class is a futile endeavor. Educators must track whether their intentions and effects on students are equitable or whether they exhibit a personal bias.

An educator should be able to say, "This student drove me nuts in how we related to each other on an interpersonal level, but they did the work and met the stated requirements of the class. Therefore, this student received high marks in the class." The same educator should also be able to say, "This student was a kind, friendly, and well-liked student who I enjoyed interacting with in class. Unfortunately, they did not meet the stated requirements of the class. Therefore, this student received below average marks in the class." Considerations should not be changed based on personal preferences or aversions to the individual student. They should not be different, for example, for the student whose parent is regularly involved in checking in on the student than they are for the student whose parents are not regularly engaged in the performance of their children in the class.

Of course, there can be variation in what a student's goals are for themselves, or a shift in the course itself that requires a change in expectations or considerations for the entire class. There should even be considerations provided for accommodations based on the needs of each student. But with all of those considerations, it is the responsibility of the educator to set and define the expectations, protocols that apply to all students, and evidence of growth that all students will be held to. If there are students that are exceptions to these expectations, an educator needs to amend the expectations for the entire class, because the expectation itself is not an equitable expectation. This may not be a reduction in rigor, but may be a more open approach to what students are able to do at the beginning of the class and what they are able to do at the end.

Some of this we, as dance educators, do as second nature, often meeting students where they are and helping them progress based on the capabilities they demonstrate in class. I suggest that instead of employing movable logic, this process should instead involve recategorizing the elements the class will be assessed on instead of thinking of differentiation as having a particular logic of assessment for one student and different logic for another student. For example, in the dance studio, the class requirement may not need to be that every student is able to successfully execute a specific skill, such as a double pirouette, or be able to execute the movement phrase switching the side of the body the phrase is done on. Rather, depending on the class, the goal may be for students to be able to clearly articulate their strengths, goals, and the efforts they have instituted to meet those goals. Other common general rubric markers include tracking a student's ability to stay focused during class; their ability to fully commit in their physical execution of movement during class time; and their improvement over time, even if the student isn't successful at executing movement phrases at the same level as the teacher has demonstrated.

Another area of behaviors that exhibit the negative effects of bias are in-group favoritism or out-group discrimination. While there are certainly structural and pervasive systems of inequity that are all too common in the classroom—ranging from socioeconomic class, to race, to gender identity—there are also a plethora of smaller personal preferences that dictate what is established as favorable and unfavorable in a program. This includes the friendly extra step a teacher may have taken in assisting a friend's child but did not take with other students. It may be justifying why you were unable to help a student who was unavailable to attend your office hours because of their work schedule, but were able to meet with the student who graduated from your old high school outside of your office hours. A student who comes from your hometown, is from the country you traveled to that is near and dear to your heart, or has a similar personality or visual look about them are all examples of potential sites of favoritism. These may feel more personal and may seem different than issues of racism, classism, and heterosexism. But ultimately when a person makes an inequitable determination or decision rather than one based on objective, explicit factors that apply to everyone, bias is often influencing the decision.

Rubrics or course content may include elements of bias not apparent to the person who developed the elements of evaluation. The elements that determine student performance can only be as inclusive as their creator has the capacity to consider. Take, for example, early childhood testing. An educator I worked with shared her frustration about Pre-K vocabulary testing. She went on to share a story of a word test where the instructor says a word, and the student explains to her what that word means. In her example, the word was "hood." The student explained that the word meant "where I live." For the student, who was living in a public housing complex steps from the school, his neighbor*hood* was a wholly appropriate answer that I argue was more contextually accurate and relevant in the student's life than the sanctioned responses. The responses that were acceptable in the testing key included the head covering on your clothing or the top of the front of a car. In the context of the definition required by the test creators, the student's answer was incorrect.

The question then becomes: where in the context of dance is a student's response in class seen as poor or inaccurate by the teacher, when in fact, the student is providing contextually appropriate and relevant answers in their own daily lives that the instructor is simply not knowledgeable or aware of? When, in an improvisation class, for example, are the prompts provided by the instructor seen as an opportunity for a student to respond with movement from a genre of dance celebrated by the student but unfamiliar to the instructor? Are these physical responses to the prompt then seen as unconnected, nongermane, or a poor embodiment of the prompt, because the student chooses to respond to the prompt in a dance genre other than modern dance? When we list a course title as "Improvisation" but do not specify a bias to any particular dance genre, how can we claim to assess students objectively with unstated assumptions about dance genres operating in the class?

An example of student alienation resulting from a teacher centering her own preferences in a performance course comes from my experience teaching at a private high school. The school had just begun to accept international students. A new international student shared with me that she was very excited about taking classes in the performing arts, including theater and dance. Her first love was theater, so she signed up for the theater improvisation class. The theater instructor began the semester with a series of improvisation prompts that were based on U.S. politics. This, by default, placed the international student, who had just arrived in the U.S. from China as a first-year high school student, at a disadvantage in the class. The theater instructor, after speaking with the student, asked if I would be able to take the student into my dance class because of the student's inability to engage in the class prompts. The irony of an improvisation class wherein the instructor was unable to improvise a set of more inclusive prompts for the class was not at all lost on me. I valued having this student in my class because her experience allowed for my own personal learning about how to become more inclusive as I integrated her into my dance class.

These examples demonstrate how implicit biases take place. For a more pointed examination of what manifestations of implicit bias look like in dance education, I have organized the ways that implicit bias shows up in dance education into observational biases, aesthetic biases, and epistemic biases. These categories are about how we see (observation), what we find artistically beautiful (aesthetics), and how we come to know and create knowledge (epistemology). In dance, observation, for example, takes place prominently in dance technique classes, but can also happen in less prominent but still significant ways in other settings—for example, observing student interactions outside of the classroom. Aesthetic biases often occur in the design and choreographic process courses and can also be significant in reviewing applicant choreography in dance auditions. Epistemic biases frequently occur in history and theory courses in a dance program. Of course, these biases can also happen in other areas in the life of a dance program, such as in consideration of guest artists for the year. Each of these categories are certainly interrelated and can overlap. The categories are a way to highlight some of the more frequent conditions for each kind of bias, though they do not dictate the only conditions under which each category of bias can show up.

Technique Courses: Biases in Observation

The observation process is riddled with opportunities for implicit biases to inform the analysis and assessment of human movement and behavior and, by extension, student performance in dance classes. Observation bias not only manifests in the dance studio, but also in movement analysis courses, in class content relating to the application of analysis and assessment in the dance studio, and in observation of students outside of class sessions. Specifically, when watching student movement in phrase work and behavior in transitions throughout the class, what Moore and Yamamoto call **body prejudices** can manifest.[15] *Body prejudice* is the projection of meaning associated with a movement from a different context onto the movement in its current or future context. Moore and Yamamoto explain,

> Like body knowledge, body prejudice originates from our capacity to categorize and generalize on the basis of personal experience. Over time, a positive or negative meaning comes to be associated with a certain type of movement. If this meaning is automatically projected onto all similar movements, regardless of context and modifying details, an inappropriate and prejudicial reaction may result.[16]

Because interpreting body language is so often an unconscious and ongoing process that intersects with aspects such as the race, body size, or the clothing of a person, it is challenging to parse what is intentionally and consciously linked to an observer's determination and what is constructed more by implicit biases and unconscious associations.

Separating out intentional and subconscious associations in interpreting human movement becomes even more difficult when the observer has constructed their interpretation based on the frame of an in-group community whose perspectives already align with the observer's perspective. This can come from a number of different groups, including dance training and education communities, fellow dancers that share the observer's aesthetic sensibilities, and cultural in-groups who have sociocultural, lived experiences that are similar to the observer. In a dance program with colleagues who have similar educational backgrounds, aesthetic preferences, education or training, and/or sociocultural backgrounds, it is increasingly more difficult to understand a divergent perspective when so much of their fellow observers' lived experiences include similar social messaging. The larger the community of observers with similar experiences, the more difficult it is for the group as a whole to value the input of an outlier when it opposes the majority's experiences and perspectives.

An example of the power of how pervasive common biases in dance affect students in a dance class is when a larger dancer does not meet the technical standards of the teacher's expectations. Sometimes this assessment is based on the student not meeting clear and explicit expectations in the class, but more often, larger students are evaluated on their body and its deviation from the physical norms in the class. Executing movement looks different on differently-shaped bodies. Thus, larger bodies often become the outlier to the standards set in a class where the majority of dancers are thinner. Another example of implicit biases manifesting in dance classes based on dominant group norms and assumptions occurs when teachers interpret a Black student's body language in between the performance of movement phrases as lazy or immature, even though it may, for some who observe the class, reflect similar the language of White students. It would be challenging to track this bias without the knowledge of implicit memories ingrained in society. These messages or implicit memories that affect observation and analysis may have a long history in the nation. In the case of the observation of Black student behavior, the history of minstrel performances and their concomitant interpretations of Black bodies may still influence the unconscious memories of the observer. The lack of familiarity with the behavior, or a lack of respect or empathy for Black people may incite the implicit aversion for Black student behavior. The systemic distance pervasive in the U.S. between Black communities and White communities results in White observers deferring to implicit memories or misrepresentations of Black culture that distort the observer's analysis of Black dance students' behavior. This can take place no matter the level of training in observation and analysis, from the novice observer to a highly trained movement analyst such as those trained in the analytical systems of Laban.

Laban Movement Analysis and Observational Bias

Laban Movement Analysis (LMA) is a system of analyzing human movement originally based on the work of Rudolf Laban.[17] It is one of a number of systems that stem from Laban's work and a long line of other contributors from the Labanotation to the Language of Dance systems developed by Dr. Hutchinson Guest. In recent history the contributions of Irmgard Bartenieff have become such a significant contribution to the work that LMA in some certification programs may also be referred to as Laban-Bartenieff Movement Analysis (LBMA) which I will use as we progress. The LBMA system has four major areas of focus: Body, Effort, Shape, and Space. "Body" considers what body part is moving or initiating movement and what connective organizing pattern of movement the body is using to move. "Effort" speaks to the quality of the movement or the inner sentiment that colors the way movement is being executed. "Shape" addresses the components of how the body forms shapes or transitions from one shape to another. "Space" addresses where the whole body or body parts orient to or travel through space. This system is an attempt to create a full, complex, and dynamic way to articulate *all* the possibilities of human movement.[18]

What systems of movement analysis like LBMA offer the field of dance education are established structures and standards that hold in place and can be consistently applied to movement encounters from person to person? When there is a standard definition of Strong Weight, for instance, deviation in different observers' assignation of Strong Weight can serve to illuminate the differences in perception between people knowledgeable about the defining features of Strong Weight. Without the standards of common language and methodology with which to relay descriptions and analysis, it would be far more challenging to pinpoint where perspectives diverge and where patterns of similarity and difference in perception occur. What a system is unable to do is to speak to the ways of seeing that exist outside of that particular paradigm of the system of movement analysis.

I recently attended a workshop with fellow Laban Movement Analysts who were dance educators certified in the Laban Movement Analysis (LMA/LBMA) systems.[19] In this workshop, there was discussion about how Laban Movement Analysts cope with and address the biases in the observation and analysis process. In the discussion, a number of Certified Movement Analysts asserted that, with practice under the guidance of more experienced analysts, bias can be reduced. This struck me as a rather curious argument. What piqued my curiosity is how we as analysts take into account the amount of social growth and awareness that has taken place since 1926, when Rudolf Laban traveled to the U.S. to later publish his experience of the racial and ethnic groups he encountered in the U.S.[20] Consider how the social messages of that time differ from today's messages. How are we to assume that those who have been conducting movement analyst observations would be able to provide a more effective analysis for today's historical context? Through further research, I found bias addressed in a similar way in the 1984 article "The Potential of Movement Analysis as a Research Tool: A Preliminary Analysis." In this article a team approach is employed that uses both the Effort/Shape and Labanotation systems[21] to reduce what the authors describe as "bias resulting from individuals' tendencies to focus only on one system, or on specific components of one of the systems, in their own educational development and research."[22]

What I know from my own personal experience as an African American, female-identifying Certified Laban-Bartenieff Movement Analyst caused me to pause and reflect on this assertion. I am enthralled with the notion of bias in the LBMA work and how the brain-body interprets what we experience in current dialogues around implicit bias. The task here is to examine and differentiate my personal understanding and analysis of implicit bias, and how that personal orientation to the term is both similar to and different from the conversations about bias I am having in the LBMA community. I assert that the discussion of bias in the movement analysis exchanges addressed above are separate and distinct from recent developments in the social sciences on how implicit bias operates in the brain-body.

In movement observation and analysis, of particular concern for the purposes of this book are the implicit biases an educator has in observing and analyzing the moving body. The implicit biases of focus for me are not tendencies to emphasize or lean toward certain aspects of the Laban systems of analysis.[23] Instead the biases I speak of are internal, sociocultural preferences for seeing the world and making meaning in particular ways that vary from one culture to another. Examples include but are not limited to biases triggered relating to visible markers of race or skin color, the size or shape of a mover's body, and other mechanisms related to sociocultural power dynamics.

I assert that the process of observation and analysis of dance and student behavior reflects two areas of implicit bias. The first is the confirmation biases of the individual observer that are based on personal experiences and prior interactions or reports about students and can also be extensions of their own previous teachers' biases. The second area of implicit bias is rooted in the areas of perception that go unnoticed within the LBMA system that are based on the cultures the LBMA system was created within over its history.

These analytical biases occur because LBMA was not developed within, and has minimal cultural connection to the diverse, multicultural landscape of dance cultures and educational contexts being analyzed in classrooms today. The student observations made under the LBMA system are a demonstration of the observer's cultural perspectives, experiences, sources of knowledge, and systematic training and interpretations of the movement, not of any particular truths inherent in the movement itself. The observation and analysis of student performance is instead a relational, collaborative endeavor in which the culture being observed—in this case, the student performances and behavior in and outside of class—demonstrates phenomena and embodied knowledge, while the other culture—the instructor observing and assessing the student—reveals its frame of reference for observation, expectations in the learning environment, and meaning-making.

Anthropologist Brenda Farnell also makes a point to articulate the value of Laban's system of notation in navigating this reorientation and dialogue between cultural perspectives.[24] She speaks of Laban's value in the context of ethnographic study of dance, but I assert it is also applicable in dance education. Farnell explains that analysis of movement is incomplete without dialogue with the mover to glean a fuller understanding of the cultural context and orientation of the mover. This more accurate analysis takes place after acquiring the observed population's—in this case, the students as individuals and the dynamics between students in the classroom—understanding of the intent and context of the movement.

With students who are learning, this can be a challenge as they explore their own language and vocabulary for movement and their own cultural practices alongside what the instructor offers as institutional knowledge or dance education standards of reference for various movement concepts. I argue there are elements in operation in dance studios and classrooms that the Laban systems of analysis may not include or consider.[25] A system can only create structures based within the cultural frame of its origin that most thoroughly affix to and articulate what movement takes place in that specific cultural frame.[26] Any elements that are not valued, attended to, or visible in the cultural frame of the viewer are invisible, misinterpreted, or devalued in the analysis process.

The interpretation of student movement and behaviors, when presented in the culture of the educator-analyst, often resonates with the dominant culture present in the dance education environment and emanates a common-sense logic already established and operating as the norm in that educational environment. This is because the educator-analyst and dominant culture often share a common cultural framework, not because the interpretation is any more true than the analysis of a different system or perspective, but rather because educators serve as gatekeepers to what systems of knowledge are deemed acceptable within their community. In the world of anthropology, ethnographers look at their analysis, description, and explanation of other cultures to become familiar with how a culture perceives the world. Within dance education, to become familiar with how a teacher perceives the world, look at their analysis, description, and explanation of students, artists, educators, and scholars. Thus, to become familiar with how a teacher perceives the world, look at their approaches to teaching and assessment of students, and their evaluations of artists and educators who are being considered for positions in the dance program. Therein lies how the teacher views, frames, and organizes both the concepts involved in the movement analysis process as well as the students themselves. The frames LBMA or the *Natyashastra*, an ancient Sanskrit compendium on the performing arts in India, provide, for example, reflect cultural constructs of German or Eurocentric perception for the former, and Indian or Southeast Asian perception for the latter. These systems say as much about the viewer and their cultural orientation in perceiving as it does the movement being analyzed.

Critical Theory: Power's Effect on Perception

Power changes perception in dance education settings. Certain biases are part of a larger cultural system of oppression and inequity. These biases are often missing or only considered in superficial ways in objective or neutral observation analysis, creative research, and scholarship in the field of dance education. Not only does quantitative social science research in implicit bias bear this inequity out, the qualitative work of critical theory also illuminates the operation of power dynamics that make bias invisible to society in general, and to students and teachers in this particular context. Critical theory creates a philosophical frame with which to track the influences of sociopolitical power dynamics on systems of culture, thought, and standards of knowledge within dance education. Pertinent to the field of dance education, the principles of critical theory call into question how neutrality and universality perpetuate systems of power.

The label "neutral" establishes a lens that asks that culturally-relative biases, expectations, and values of the so-called "neutral" party be disregarded or deemed invisible in studio and classroom learning and assessment. This neutral party often gets to establish this norm because of its social in-group or dominant status in society. In the classroom the educator has a dominant status compared to that of a student. Intersections, however, between other identity markers and power dynamics can make the simple construct of teacher as dominant and students as subordinate more complex. There are studies, for example, of how majority White student classes can provide damaging course evaluations to educators of color or female-identifying educators thereby putting their teaching performance evaluations at risk. To employ the mask of neutrality or objectivity, an instructor asks those who receive their analyses to remove the effects that their personal experiences have on how they construct meaning and value. I illustrate an example of this implausibility in this excerpt:

> An assessment I received in a Laban Movement Analysis session included a description of my engagement at the beginning of the process. One instructor paused and held up both hands in front of her, palms down with flexed wrists angling her fingers toward the ground, a gesture often used to depict an animal's paws. She quickly nodded her head up and down as if to make reference to the excited panting of a puppy. She landed on the word "childlike" to describe my eagerness to learn. My evaluators continued using the words "lazy" and "unenthusiastic" to describe my initial disposition […] The paradoxical feedback of being essentially childlike and lazy put be in mind of the stereotypes of Black people established in the minstrel shows of the 1800s.[27]

In this assessment example from a learning environment, the assumption of neutrality on the part of the instructor is a damaging one. Without the context of understanding that educators raised in the U.S. are exposed to social messaging of Black people being both lazy and childlike, the two paradoxical notions applied to my performance might seem nonsensical. But contextualizing the integration of both eagerness and a lack of enthusiasm within a social structure that simultaneously has projected *childlike* and *lazy* onto Black bodies for hundreds of years, these tropes begin to illuminate the logic of racism underlying the assessment of my performance. Neutrality insinuates that no such contextual history applies and that there is only the reality spoken into existence by the educator-analyst.

The notion of universality is equally problematic because it establishes the defining features of an insider-outsider boundary of acceptance. This boundary is established by assigning everything that applies to the *universal* standard as normative, and that everything does not apply as an outlier or substandard. In the field of dance, I concede that the grandiosity of the search to articulate what is universal about movement continues to inspire movement principles, theories, and discoveries about the moving body all over the world. This examination is a valuable question that generates meaningful knowledge about the moving body. What is crucial is remembering that *universal* is a lowercase word. Principles are only universal in that they provide culturally specific answers that apply in broad ways within each community as that community explores the defining features of universality for their collective experience. The moment we deem some element of movement Universal with a capital "U," a TRUTH that applies to all cultures, we immediately exclude individuals and/or groups who do not adhere or concede to those defining qualifications. By extension, those who do not fit into the universal standard are judged as deficient or belonging to some category of *other*. The foundations upon which the justification for Western intervention and colonization are built include assertions that dance researchers are neutral. These research findings promote cultural structures, principles, and behaviors of the West asserting they should be universal standards. Both universality and neutrality, in the context of the United States, function as a way to normalize the values, biases, and expectations established by way of colonialism that serve to benefit heteronormative White males.[28] In actuality, these assertions are a global ruse that privilege and center the norms of White males all over the planet.

This also applies in the aesthetic application and categorization of dance within dance education. The categories of social dance, Western dance, world dance, modern dance, contemporary dance, popular dance, concert dance, and vernacular dance are merely one perspective within which to organize a broad range of dance forms. I know in the fields of dance and dance education we lean on these categories to help students understand what to expect in dance classes they are taking. We dance educators, as those with the privilege to name, restructure, and be responsive to new systems of knowledge, can initiate change. Dance educators can interrogate these categories and restructure courses to address power inequities present in these terms, include diverse student perspectives in these critical discussions for their experiences of power inequity in courses, and challenge students to take risks in enrolling in newly named and newly structured courses with explanations of how these changes speak to systemic inequity.

I remember choreographing what for me was a modern dance work to a Stevie Wonder song in college. It included modern dance vocabulary and intentionally flowed between rhythmic phrasing with and against the music. When I showed the work to my professor, she shared how, for her, the work was a jazz dance piece. I wondered if this perception was primarily triggered by the aesthetic of the work or that a Black body was performing the work. With no discussion of intentional choreographic design or aesthetic choices based on modern dance tenets, what the professor observed is not enough to determine as a final word what genre the dance work is in. An implicit racial bias could have been in operation with this professor who was also a Certified Movement Analyst in her categorization of my work. Without a fuller conversation held between us about this disconnect, how we both interpreted the dance is a missed opportunity for mutual understanding.

The importance of articulating the meaning of implicit bias and how it is applied in the Laban analysis community has significant effects in application of the Laban systems. Clarifying the difference between conceptual biases articulated within the system and implicit biases in the perception and meaning-making process of the analysts as they observe and analyze movement is an important distinction for dance studios and classrooms. I focus on the latter: how the mind categorizes new experiences and correlates them to implicit memories and biases held by the perceiver. Attending to the mind's unconscious correlating, sorting, and eliminating of details during an experiential movement event is significant because it helps us better understand the analytical findings of that lived movement experience. Understanding how the mind processes information in a way that supports its current beliefs, biases, and experiences calls into question the notions of positivist, "neutral" analysis, evaluation, and assessment in the classrooms and studios of dance programs. The effects of adhering to the narratives and cultural contexts of those deemed experts in the field or those who align with perceptions of culturally dominant norms is an exclusionary orientation that restricts the growth, development, empathetic capacity, memory, and inter-relational dialogue between educators as observers and assessors of dance and the communities that are the subjects of their assessments.

Training an educator-analyst to see the world through the pre-established frame of Laban's theories and principles illuminates all of the aspects of the system and in so doing makes invisible other aspects that are not part of the system's frame. For example, in the ancient Indian performance treatise, the *Natyashastra*, aesthetics are categorized by the elements of bhava that dancers convey and rasa that audiences feel.[29] Because these are not elements of the LBMA system, they are not used as a frame in LBMA and thus not seen by an observer who has not been introduced to the elements of bhava and rasa.

In addressing these negative effects of implicit bias, I offer a different perspective on how movement analysis systems can be used across cultures, an approach that promotes dialogue between LBMA and other perspectives on movement as a way to decenter LBMA as a universal or

4. Biases and Behaviors 107

even central approach for analysis. Laban analysis systems benefit from testing their boundaries through application in cultural contexts, like diverse classrooms and studios, that do not organize an understanding of dance through the elements of Laban systems. Laban systems can enrich their understanding of their own concepts and understand the systems' connections and differences from other perspectives if it also concedes to being one of many ways to see and analyze movement. Acknowledging the truths and frames of understanding movement and dance in cultures outside of Laban's Western-centered perspective can be a rich way to better understand how very culturally specific the frame of Laban analysis systems are. This shift in perspective helps establish a deeper understanding of how Laban systems align with the Western world and how that orientation differs from the frames of a myriad of complex and intersecting cultures a teacher finds in dance studios and classrooms. To progress a step further, understanding the power structures that centered Laban's work and marginalized the analysis of others helps discern where the value of the system is most applicable—within a predominantly White Western concert dance context—and most harmful—when applied as a definitive truth to marginalized non-Western dance contexts.

Solutions to disrupting implicit biases in dance education involve personal, inter-relational, and systemic approaches, which I illustrate from my own personal ethnographic approach later in Chapter 5. Examining the role implicit bias plays in each of these areas—personal, inter-relational, and systemic—has the potential to deepen the educator-analyst's understanding of their own implicit biases. This examination can also strengthen relationships between educators and their students and colleagues and disrupt the implicit assumptions of universality, objectivity, and neutrality present in Laban analysis systems. Disrupting the negative effects of implicit biases in Laban analysis systems has the potential to create space for critical, rigorous dialogue between those within the Laban systems and introduce knowledge from students and prospective colleagues with expertise as cultural insiders to other ways of understanding, observing, and analyzing movement and dance forms. While disruption can feel chaotic and uncomfortable, the potential for change that is deep and broad in the movement analysis community is worth the exploration.

Moore and Yamamoto continue to unpack the observation and analysis process by offering ideas of what reduces the level of difference in movement meaning between the mover(s) and the observer-analyst. In the case of the dance education setting, the observer assigned the role of analyzing movement is most often the instructor, and the students are most often the movers being observed. Of course, this process does also apply to instances in the dance studio wherein students learn how to analyze movement by observing others under the guidance of teacher feedback or observe the instructor for clarity in the content being taught. Moore and Yamamoto's solutions include clear movement; acuity of observation; similar sociocultural backgrounds and personal familiarity of movers and observers; and an observer's strong desire to understand.[30] I am less interested in reducing the level of divergence between mover and observer here, and more interested in the clarity with which the mover and observer can explicitly communicate context, perspective, and the correlating evidence of their own perspective. Exchanges where discussions distinguish and articulate differences between analytical perspectives is where parsing out explicit biases and implicit biases can be productive. The greater the ability to articulate personal biases and track the cultural structures and orientations that support them, the greater the potential for the vulnerability of exchange and discovery through dialogue.

The need for established criteria and standards in organizing concepts and aspects of movement are a clear reason why movement observation systems are useful in helping to diminish implicit bias. Banaji and Greenwald include evidence-based guidelines, criteria, and structures as a tool in disrupting implicit bias *blind spots*.[31] Applying a structured system to the movement observation process is a way to track the presence of assumptions, biases, and divergent thinking in the analysis of observers. What is key in the context of sociopolitical power dynamics that often play out on a global scale in cross-cultural studio and classroom settings, however, is that one system of analysis is not applied universally. No system is completely universal, neutral, or unbiased, and rather should be understood as a culturally specific lens. Contextualizing each system's lens and positionality is essential to help understand the operation and framework of that system for students.

For this reason, it is crucial that the observer abandon the notion of neutrality if cultural proximity and familiarity with the mover(s) being observed is a requirement. Before classroom assessment, the observer should establish their cultural proximity and positionality to the performance so students can understand assessments generated by the observer's analysis. The student being observed would then be able to read the resulting research findings with an informed understanding of how the observer-analyst is making sense of their movement and culture. Clarity of movement and acuity of observation are both culturally specific. What is clear in one person's mind may not be clear to another person. Even through the lens of LMA for example, we know there can be clarity of body part articulation in a movement, while there is simultaneously an unclear spatiality. We know one analyst can discern Effort dynamics, for example, while being less sensitive to Shaping. The level of movement clarity or observational acuity in the classroom also depends on the purpose of the observation. The detail required for feedback in a repertory class, where students must perform the dance work to nuanced specifications, is different from the feedback required in a Laban analysis class where students are improvising an Effort movement prompt.

Creative and Performance Process Courses: Biases in Aesthetics

In classes that are built around student creativity or design such as creative process, composition, choreographic design, and improvisation, there is another way implicit biases can negatively affect equitable assessment in the classroom. While all of the negative effects of implicit bias from the observation section above can also manifest in these settings, the additional category of aesthetic bias can also materialize. As articulated in Chapter 1, there is an established systemic power dynamic in what aesthetic orientation educational institutions, presenters, critics, and funders determine to have *aesthetic value*. There are also the aesthetic biases of each individual educator and how it affects observation, assessment, and evaluation in classes geared towards students developing their own creative work. In these classes, it is difficult to avoid centering one's own aesthetic values in the class. For this reason, steps should be taken to decenter the instructor's aesthetic biases in order to support the growth, development, and articulation of student aesthetic sensibilities.

When educators require students to explore the creative processes attuned to only the aesthetic choices of the instructor, they are essentially molding student sensibilities to the standards established by the instructor. In this way, the creative process becomes a replication of existing systems rather than a wholly unique, creative journey for students. The imposition of teacher choreographic ideas or aesthetic affinities, particularly when they are presented as *the* process or perspective instead of *a* process or perspective, stifles student innovation, as well as student voice, perspective, agency, and creativity. It shifts the creative process into a repetition of existing mechanistic and formulaic processes, a problematic endeavor if the process is presented as the standard structure for dance creation.

In classes where students are creating their own dance works or designing their own creative content, it is important that the teacher be intentional in subverting their own personal likes and dislikes, or else teachers should be explicit in stating that students will be assessed based on the personal sensibilities of the instructor. One way to do this is to establish a clear rubric of what you are considering in the assessment and what you are not. Be explicit about what you are "grading" about the work. Are you grading the student commitment to their own working process? If so, what does evidence of commitment look like for you as the teacher? If you are grading the quality of the final product, this is a rich site for a teacher's aesthetic biases to manifest. To decenter teacher bias, students could assess the final products of their classmates based on the rubric created by the teacher. In advanced level courses where students have already created work on their own, the rubric could be developed by the student so that the aesthetic frame is set by the student, not by the teacher or by some other external measure. It is important to examine as a teacher the *quality* of the work. If there is an established standard in the culture of your curriculum or dance program, it is necessary to explicitly name that aesthetic orientation. This then gives students a way to both attune to the expectations of the course while also allowing them to negotiate how they can include and incorporate their own perspectives and aesthetic biases into their work. If there is a student who is working in a style or genre unfamiliar to you as the teacher, it is imperative to include an external eye on the work that is able to see the work through the aesthetic lens of the dance genre instead of the lens of the teacher's sensibilities. This can be done through incorporating guest artists as evaluators or even including members of student groups on campus who specialize in that dance genre. Inviting students from school dance groups has the added benefit of incorporating students who may not be involved in the course as acknowledged experts of dance forms in which the instructor is not well versed.

Theory Courses: Biases in Epistemology

Theory and writing courses in dance programs can also involve the above-mentioned markers of implicit bias in the classroom. Observation of how a student sits, listens, takes notes, and communicates in class can be a site of implicit bias or body prejudice. The choices of dance content (i.e., dance clips, performances, dance companies, etc.) or the dismissal of or disregard for student contributions to examples of dance content demonstrate aesthetic bias. It is not enough as an educator to hold fast to the assertion that these are the dance works that I know. It is crucial that dance content include a variety of diverse examples that align with the concepts the teacher is illustrating, not on the preferences for dance works the teacher has.

In recent years, a number of online dance educator groups have developed via social media platforms for dance educators to exchange

4. Biases and Behaviors 111

resources from their areas of expertise. These can be helpful sites for finding resources for a particular class topic. An additional consideration in teaching theory courses such as dance appreciation, dance history, movement theory, and movement analysis, etc., is the impact of **epistemic bias**. *Epistemic bias* is the preference for or aversion to certain knowledge systems. For example, in the field of dance, there is a common understanding or perspective that non-dancers do not value the knowledge that comes from bodily movement and instead privilege written work as knowledge. Another way to understand this statement is that non-dancers tend to have an epistemic bias for written knowledge as valid and an aversion to embodied knowledge systems, thinking of them as non-valid resources for knowledge.

There are several ways that epistemic bias results in exclusionary practices in the classroom. Holroyd and Puddifoot articulate a number of these sites of injustice in their work.[32] There is the bias of who a person considers a reputable, credible source of knowledge, a bias the authors classify as a **testimonial injustice**. If a teacher determines that content from social media outlets, for example, are not acceptable simply because it has been sourced from social media, this is a testimonial bias the teacher has.

Another epistemic bias is the determination of who gets to be an expert on dance forms that are not from their cultural background. It is a common occurrence in the field of dance that dancers and scholars who study a form that is not from their own cultural background end up teaching that dance form. The idea of a dancer or dance scholar being identified as an expert of a dance that is not from their cultural background is common. The power dynamics of a dancer who has no cultural relationship to a dance form being designated as an expert of that dance form is a phenomenon identified as "**epistemic appropriation injustice**" by Holroyd and Puddifoot.[33] I personally have been asked to teach a number of dance forms not from my cultural background, including West African dance, Latin dance forms, and Indian dance forms. I share the problematic and precarious nature of this predicament with my students so that they can consider their approach in their own dance careers. I also bring in experts in the forms, and when students have expertise or cultural knowledge they would like to share about the dance form, I include space for students to share as a knowledge source.

Epistemic exploitation is another injustice linked to implicit bias. In this instance, the cultural insider of a marginalized or disenfranchised group is asked to do the additional labor of explaining the dynamics, nature, and lived experience of their oppression in order for those of the dominant culture to educate themselves on the matter with no compensation for sharing their knowledge. An example that illuminates and distinguishes epistemic exploitation from epistemic appropriation would be if I as a cultural outsider accepted a job teaching a West African dance class (epistemic appropriation), then asked a cultural insider and expert West African dancer colleague to help explain concepts of the dance form to me for free (epistemic exploitation). This not only diminishes the value of the expertise and labor of the disenfranchised person, but it also adds additional work the expert is not acknowledged for or compensated for doing. There is also the added emotional labor of having to share difficult dynamics of oppression for the benefit of those implicated in that oppression.

Hermeneutic injustice is a bias that addresses the privilege embedded in canonized content, including writing resources, dance works, artists, and scholars that are present in standard curriculum. This bias calls into question why the performers, scholars, and the content of the standardized reference points are standard in the dance field. Why has some content fallen into obscurity, while other content remains at the center of common-use content? For example, in a number of dance history curricula Ruth St. Denis, a White woman dancer, is referenced in more depth and with more frequency than Pearl Primus, a Black woman dancer and anthropologist, when both made notable contributions to the study of dances outside of a particular culture.

Finally, there is **contributory injustice**. The bias of contributory injustice privileges the connection or affirmation of the dance education community and academic publishing platforms in order for content to be acceptable in academic research. It is a bias about what is appropriate and what is not appropriate to source as citation material. Similar to biases in canon content selection, this speaks to what resource materials are privileged in dance scholarship beyond the canon. This bias often couples with the hermeneutic bias of what is in the canon, because there is a common assumption that the examples and citations referenced by a course are the appropriate models for citation by students or contemporaries in the field. Contributory injustice refers to a bias for certain resources that are deemed acceptable to cite and thus often replicates the use of dance canon and, by extension, justifies that canon's presence in dance curricula. An example of this comes from my own personal choices for citations in my writing. I received feedback in a peer review submission that referencing the work of Maxine Greene was problematic, because she is a dated source. Why is Greene's (1917–2014) work considered dated for discussions in the field of dance education while John Dewey's (1859–1952) work stands the test of time in terms of being an acceptable reference in dance education publications? Who determines which sources stand the test of time, and which do not? In classrooms, this could involve, for example, a student not being able to use Beyoncé as a dance reference in a research paper, because she is a dance performer from the popular dance arena, not from the concert dance community.

While there may be a number of other ways that implicit bias manifests in dance education, this is an initial attempt to lay out methods to articulate, categorize, and engage in discussions about how implicit biases manifest in dance education. For example, at my current status in higher education, I have little lived experience with how these manifestations of implicit bias may show up in administrative environments beyond the reach of my untenured, junior faculty status. There are more senior, experienced faculty that could speak to manifestations witnessed in their responsibilities as tenured faculty. Further, as a member of Generation X, I also have less experience with how growing up with access to technology and social media affect how biases manifest for my contemporaries in the field. For example, I know there is research done on how human biases affect search algorithms and other forms of technological design.[34] This certainly can be a rich site for further discussion in the context of how those immersed in online dance platforms experience forms of implicit bias. I assert that this is not at all an exhaustive list of ways to talk about and illuminate how implicit biases show up in dance education, and thus invite you to entertain other ways to talk about and organize these manifestations.

ACTIVITY BOX #13: Bias Superlatives

After reviewing the various ways that implicit bias manifests as detailed in this chapter, think about your own personal experiences in dance education and how these manifestations of biases might have been operating. Think about two instances you feel implicit biases were in operation, and name the superlative of the manifestation of bias. For example, was it the oddest, the worst, the most humorous, the most physically demanding, the itchiest, or the least physically demanding? After assigning the superlative category for the examples, take a moment to journal about why you chose that superlative. If there is time, feel free to explore if you can pinpoint an opposing superlative example. For instance, if you labeled one event the most physically demanding, can you identify an event that was the least physically demanding example of that same form of implicit bias? Take a moment to read over and reflect on anything you notice about what you have described.

5

Feeders and Disruptors of Bias

In Chapter 4, I explain how implicit biases show up in a number of ways in dance education. The first part of this chapter is dedicated to describing the elements that trigger, enhance, or increase the likelihood that implicit biases affect thoughts and behaviors within dance education settings. Then, the second part of the chapter illuminates elements that disrupt the influence of implicit biases in dance education.

The feeders of implicit biases are myriad and can be as contextually complex as the manifestations of implicit bias themselves. The first, and my personal favorite, feeder of implicit bias already mentioned in Chapter 4 is "**cognitive busyness.**" It still causes me to giggle when I think about first reading about the concept in Levinson's work and how the description jumped out at me as a great description of teaching.[1] He describes *cognitive busyness* in the following way: "Studies on the influence of 'cognitive busyness' on stereotypes and false memories indicate that people generate even more false memories when they are under stress, distracted, older, or otherwise cognitively busy."[2] Another factor that influences the cognitive load is if there is a time or speed element to the activity. As I read this description, I remember thinking to myself, "Well, then, I think you just described teaching perfectly, teaching dance even more precisely." I thought of having to be mindful of keeping the pace of a class to cover an ample amount of material, noticing social interactions or behaviors that are informing the dynamics of how students are engaging in class, the stress of ensuring I am successfully relaying the necessary information students need to accomplish the goals of the class and if not how to modify my methods. All of these things are happening simultaneously on an individual student level, as well as on a larger group level. The cognitive load or cognitive busyness in teaching dance is particularly demanding.

Situations teaching dance are more prone to being influenced by implicit bias when a person is fatigued, distracted, or does not have adequate information to make an informed decision.[3] These types of environmental factors are often conditions that a dance educator cannot entirely control. Imagine the all-too-common circumstance that an educator was up late grading work or providing support for late-night rehearsals or performances. In a classroom the next day, the educator sees an interaction that was related to three other instances that the educator missed while working with other students in the class, or that happened in the previous class before students entered the classroom. Imagine the educator witnesses this interaction happening off to the side in a studio setting while the educator is leading a movement activity and keeping meticulous records of class participation or some other element of an in-class activity. Educators do this all while being mindful of staying on track with the timed guidelines of the class session and the time dedicated to that specific activity in their planning. In this common, day-in-the-life scenario of the classroom or studio, the educator is meeting each aspect of the listed factors, excluding age, involved in cognitive busyness that lend themselves to the influences of implicit biases. So, there are a number of factors to consider in order to minimize how implicit biases operate in the dance studios and classrooms. Many of these factors, however, cannot be fully controlled.

In addition to cognitive busyness, a lack of awareness of implicit biases allows the implicit biases to remain in place. This lack of awareness is often only apparent once the unconscious bias is brought into the light of conscious awareness. An example of this happened in a formal observation at a high school where I was teaching. The observer shared with me that she noted who I called on during class discussion and who I did not. In tracking my facilitation of the discussion, she shared with me that I called far more frequently on male-identifying students than on the female-identifying students in the class. I had no mechanism in place to track this behavior or tendency. Without having another set of eyes in the room to track the things I, while managing all the elements of facilitating learning, missed, I would have missed this biased tendency.

But then what to do after discovering such bias? Implicit biases can exist both simultaneously and apart from the explicit biases and beliefs operating at the surface of conscious, intentional beliefs. Once these biases float to the surface of awareness, to deny, ignore them, explain, or excuse them away as non-existent only reifies the effects of the bias, ensuring the implicit bias remains operational. Creating or developing excuses about why it isn't a bias, or explaining it away with some circumstances that warranted the behavior, assumption, or decision is unproductive to upending the bias. Of course, every situation is different in how best to tackle the work of addressing the bias. What is important is owning and reflecting on what might be disconcerting and uncomfortable ideologies that are anathema to the conscious mind and perspective but still exist beneath the surface of consciousness. This discomfort is the cognitive dissonance explained in the Introduction.

As an example on how to move forward once an implicit bias is determined, I return back to my high school gender bias example. This is one example of how to address an implicit bias head on. Once my fellow educator brought to my attention this bias of calling on the male-identified students in the class, I then sat in a reflective process. I evaluated what was happening internally that may have warranted such biased behavior. Because I had a good working relationship with the students in the class, I communicated to the class the following week what my colleague discovered from their observation. I explained to them a bit about how the benefit of observations is that I get to learn how to be better in my teaching practice. To that end, I explained that through the observation, it had been brought to my attention that I had not been calling on the female students as frequently as the male students, and that there would be a change in the class of me calling more frequently on female students in the class. I then shared that this was because it is important to hear from everyone in the class, and if this change felt uncomfortable in any way that they could come to me to propose a different way of conducting class discussions.

Determine Your Implicit Biases

To combat implicit bias, there are a number of strategies that a teacher or dance program can implement. The first is doing the work of unpacking implicit biases. This involves ascertaining your biases, then researching the exclusionary, racist, and hegemonic socialization the U.S. is mired in. This discovery and reflection process is a critical way to reframe and make visible the effects of implicit biases in dance education settings.

A starting point to determining implicit biases is to take Implicit Association Tests (IAT). These tests exploit the mind's inability to counter implicit biases when having to concentrate on several elements under a stressful time restraint, i.e., creating a cognitively busy environment. In these timed tests, where reflex is the order of the day in making various selections, when the test does not align with an implicitly held belief (for example, flowers are liked, and bugs are disliked), there will be more errors in completing the tasks and/or the test will take longer when the item on the test does not align with your implicit orientations (for example, selecting a pairing of pleasant words when they are coupled with

5. Feeders and Disruptors of Bias 117

images of bugs). In the flower-and-bug example mentioned above, if a person is asked to associate positive words with the bugs and negative words with the flowers, the majority of people who take the test struggle to complete the task on time and select answers they did not intend to choose after looking back over their answers.[4]

Harvard's *Project Implicit* study is a valuable resource in unpacking explicit and implicit biases. This online IAT measures the test subject's subconscious biases in a variety of areas such as race, ability, and weight or size. The test is designed using split-second selections to determine whether participants find association, for example, of a heavier person with positive descriptors easy or difficult. This is an online test platform, free to the public that I highly recommend taking, as it makes visible the implicit biases we have relating to varying populations of people. What is significant about this work in the field of dance is that it illuminates how the split-second observing, moving, and analyzing done in dance studios and dance classrooms can be flawed based on the subconscious or implicit biases operating before the analytical brain gains access to the sensory stimuli that trigger the effects of the implicit bias. IATs can be guides to help understand and disrupt the way in which dance is seen and perceived based on messages from socialization.

Of course, after taking the various tests, the question arises of what to do with the biases after knowing that they exist? One of the most efficacious places to start dismantling biases is to begin by sitting in the relative truth of the personal values and beliefs that are already consciously known. So much of how humans organize the world is employed by acting on the beliefs a person can name, rather than reflecting on the nature or foundation of how those beliefs came to be beliefs. Therefore, the task is to sever the attachment to thinking of beliefs as unbiased, objective truths that are foundational or operational in the discernment of dance. The arts are built on bias: the biases of artists, audiences, reviewers, certain moments in history, communities, etc. Dance in particular, with its ephemeral quality and its capacity to function apart from language or still images and objects, is so much about the preferences and detestations, the yearnings and aversions, in that moment the experiencer encounters the dance. Whether the experiencer is the mover or viewer, the lived experiences of the experiencer formulate a felt sense, even if that sentiment is boredom or contentment. Why deny that dance is very much about feeling or doing something whether that be a sensation where one is drawn to and relishes, repelled by and despises, or some other felt sense in encountering dance?

Dancers and dance educators must get to a place where they can simply speak the truth of what their biases are. Can we say out loud realities that are operational like "I prefer and have a passion for modern dance. While I like the idea of having the power to temporarily exhibit or display other dance forms on my own terms, I do not believe other dance forms should be raised to the level of appreciation, attention, and use of resources as modern dance for the following reasons…"? Can we say, "My income and career status are more important to me than giving up my position to create opportunity for a qualified dancer or educator that is underrepresented in the field and/or historically marginalized in society. Besides, in the systemically unjust environment I work in, I'm not sure having an underrepresented or historically marginalized person in the job would help much." Or "The opportunity to offer a position to a person with similar interests or backgrounds to mine feels safer and is, thus, more important to me than taking the risk I perceive of giving a person I am unfamiliar with a position." Are you willing to state plainly, "I prefer the benefit of the power I hold as an expert and influencer in the field more than relinquishing that power to disenfranchised members of the dance field"? Or "I value supporting the stability and familiarity of aesthetics found in well-established White artists in the field over the risky innovation and perspective that marginalized artists bring to the field of dance and dance education." Can you proclaim, "I value my personal power and privilege more than I value supporting, including, or hiring artists whose aesthetics are personally unfamiliar or unappealing to me"? Will you be able to say aloud, "I have less empathy and interest in supporting artists who I do not personally identify with, as it relates to my own interpersonal biases and assumptions of 'professional' behavior"? Is it possible that the lived experiences of the choreography or creative process teacher may result in a different truth about the nature and structure (or lack thereof) of creating dances than the lived experiences and working processes of their students? If so, is there space in the classroom to hold this dialogic wherein the student may engage in divergent thinking in their own personal creative process that may not align with that of the instructor?

These explicit declarations do not have to be statements that feel honorable or even feel consistent with your sense of self. They may not even be fully realized without some tracking and reflection on internal feelings and what may feel like intuitive decisions in educational deliberations and planning. Remember that the brain is capable of holding conflicting beliefs, some operating explicitly and some operating implicitly. If these sentiments run counter to how you perceive yourself to be, facing these beliefs, unpacking them, and making different, more intentional and thoughtful choices in behavior are a way to reckon with these beliefs and bring your implicit disposition more in line with how you think of yourself. It is the practice in the metaphor that Daniel Sloss sets up in the

Introduction of speaking with your Nigel to review, clean out, and resort those beliefs in the brain's rolodex of opinions.

To be able to name personal biases on the hard questions—on personal values around the access and proximity to power structures in the field or organization; on any assignation of value to various dance forms, pedagogical styles, and historically marginalized bodies and cultures; on personal capacity to hear and accept a hard truth in a moment of a bias-oriented offense or shortfall—is valuable. I recommend creating a practice of listing personal biases, aversions, and priorities. Can you rank them? Under what circumstances might they change positions on the list of priority? As you collect these biases, track decisions, behaviors, language, and thoughts that either confirm or conflict with the stated bias. Where are you in alignment with your stated biases? At what moments are you in misalignment, wherein your decisions, behaviors, language or thought are not consistent with the stated bias? This process is ripe with the potential for discovery, a moment to transition an implicit cognitive moment into an explicit realization.

One practice I integrate into my course introductions is that I clarify for students my positionality and biases as they relate to the metacognitive goals of the class. In addition to the goals of delivering course content, I share with students the cognitive, interpersonal goals I would like them to leave class having strengthened. While these tend to show up in the hidden curriculum,[5] I share with students what type of thinker, learner, and community member I would like the students to attune to for the duration of my class. For instance, I share in age-appropriate ways in my teaching environments that I affine with critical thinkers who ask the "Yes, but..." questions during class. I encourage students to push back on the knowledge that I relay or that is communicated through resource materials in the class with resources and examples from their lived experiences and own systems of knowledge.

As a dance instructor, program, studio business, or organization, once these critical and clarifying discussions have taken place, the next question is how to meet the institutional needs of the dance education goals while still addressing the cycle of oppression issues that arise in most every facet of student experience. For example, if your institution is well-resourced and highly sought-after with far more applicants wanting to attend than the institution can handle, of course there will be use of the resources to ensure that the students accepted are in line with the intentions and goals of the organization. After considering institutional goals and focus, next to consider is the evidence of how the cycle of oppression is supported, upheld, reified by the organization. For example, does the representation of the student or faculty population accurately represent the demographic information of the community being served? What is the benchmark of equitable demographic representation the organization adheres to in order to ensure a level of equitable representation within the program, business, or institution?

This line of questioning and examination leads to another aspect that buttresses implicit biases. A lack of clear standards, criteria, and rubrics feed implicit biases. What you discover in your personal implicit biases as an educator, or in your collective biases as an educational community relates and often shows up in the standards, guiding phrases, criteria, selection guidelines, and assessment rubrics of a course or program. This applies as much to the explicit biases as to the implicit ones. Your educational goals as a community should be consistent with what you explicitly state as your values and biases in your defining and identifying features.

Unfortunately, it is also often evident what implicit biases are operating when examining these sets of standards, guidelines, principles, and criteria. For example, if your dance studio is defined as a creative movement studio that celebrates all types of movers, and offers general dance classes that are not defined by the genre or style of dance, these course offerings align with your explicit bias. This bias favors creative movement and the development of improvisational and choreographic skills for students instead of training students in a specific technical form of dance. But instituting a sliding scale for class payment that requires guardians to submit their tax returns or pay stubs for confirmation without consideration for those who do not receive those forms of documentation, displays an implicit bias for those adults in the community who work jobs that provide such payment documentation. This policy excludes families from disenfranchised economic employment like low-wage or undocumented employment who do not work in jobs with such documentation and do not have financial resources for accountants that can provide proof of income for access to the studio's classes. For this reason, the more clearly an individual educator and their institutions can articulate not only their explicit values but also examine where policies, guidelines, and standards conflict with those explicit values is a significant deterrent to implicit bias.

Establishing clear rubrics that hold the educator and the dance program accountable to what they are actually looking for from students is crucial in disrupting the effects of implicit bias. Making rubrics and detailed expectations available to students and helping students understand the lens through which you are evaluating class activities helps diminish the effects of implicit bias in the observation and assessment of student performance in the studio and classroom. It also helps students communicate and have a deeper understanding of the expectations in the class. It gives students the opportunity to self-assess and to attune to the explicit expectations of the instructor, to see through the eyes of the instructor. Attuning and understanding the perspective of others is not only an effective way to help students have more agency over their own growth and development, but also a way to forge interpersonal connections and a shared frame of reference that helps students understand where they can actually be more expansive and creative in exploring new ideas for themselves.

Not only should the standards be clearly articulated, but they must also be consistently applied. These criteria must be able to apply for each student, applicant, employee, or colleague. If in the review process there is an outlier applicant that inspires the thought that there be some sort of exception to the rule or standards, it is a valuable moment to examine the potential operation of unspoken bias. An exception to the rule is a determinant that the rule or standard does not include the experiences of the out-group applicant or apply in an equitable way to all who are under consideration, whether that is in including or excluding an applicant. It is also evidence that the standards must be amended so that they can be applied to everyone. For example, what is your policy for students who cannot afford to travel to an in-person audition? Is there a different policy for domestic students around the expectation they attend an in-person audition, or is that policy the same for international students? How does the policy apply equitably for international applicants, low-income applicants, or applicants who have some other circumstance that results in prohibitive travel circumstances? How do those policies either adhere to or run counter to your explicit mission, goals, and stated identity as a program?

For dance programs, discussions held by educators and administrators about auditions and how to structure selection processes can begin at the very start of the process. Why is an audition or selection process needed for a dance program? Does your institution specialize in a particular genre that requires previous training in that particular form? How does a program reckon with the socially constructed biases the applicants carry that the program is inherently better if it is difficult to get into? Is there an abundance of applicants for which the program is unable to support the anticipated enrollment? Are the factors supporting the reasoning for auditions based on elements of elitism, scarcity of resources, or a no-longer applicable precedent—i.e., "This is the way we have always done it, though we are unsure of why"?

It is important to consider the decision to include or exclude students once the program evaluates the detrimental effects of the cycle of oppression on students. Including some students in the program while excluding others is a prevalent structure of the cycle of oppression in its most toxic application. Of course, in a perfect world all students interested in studying dance would be able to access the educational setting of their choice. Excluding some students from a dance program is a structure oriented toward social dominance orientation (SDO) in its most seemingly harmless: "But I'm just supporting those I am most familiar with, who I know or have something in common with." It is crucial to frequently and critically review whether auditions are necessary for the structural needs of the educational program. Dance programs should determine if auditions are offered in a way that risks in-group/out-group discriminatory decisions or contributes to systems of oppression. The process of auditions also opens the program up to missed opportunities to accept talented applicants when program instructors and gatekeepers make decisions affected by their implicit biases that ultimately hurt the program by steering away talent the selectors miss.[6] I have seen students with no prior training, through passion and persistence, excel at keeping up with the years of technical training that other students have had. Part of the reflection process in extending an offer to a student with less technical training is how, in an educational program, do you equitably support students and provide resources for their success? Is there reservation about the amount of time, effort, and resource a student with minimal technical training will need, while time, effort, and resource support flows freely toward exceptional students in the program? These are issues to consider and explore programmatically.

The next feeder of bias requires a level of reflection on the dynamics of power and privilege in relationships with applicants and organizations and the financial or status benefits to the educator or organization. Implicit bias thrives on there being some level of benefit for a person to engage in the bias. Take, for example, a wealthy donor who has a child applying to your dance program. Accepting the donor's child may result in financial benefit to the dance program. This benefit or privilege can affect the deliberation of potential applicants causing an unjustly favorable bias toward accepting the donor's child. Tracking the benefits, whether intended or inadvertent, of decisions, behaviors, or language used is a key component of preventing the negative effects of bias from seeping into those deliberations of a dance education community that purport to be objective and unencumbered by such considerations or benefits.

For this reason, after the standards, criteria, and rubrics have been employed, it is also crucial to track the results of evaluations to identify any potential evidence of other implicit biases. Not tracking the results of these deliberation processes is another reinforcer of implicit bias. Just as my observation example about gender bias in Chapter 4 tracked the students called upon in class, devising ways in which to analyze the results of choices, decisions, or actions that take place is a way to illuminate evidence of implicit biases.

Changes in policies and protocols can deter bias from influencing decisions, if well-designed, quantitative evidence-based data tracks the reduction of hidden biases at the administrative level. My contribution to countering these implicit biases in the work as dance educators involves developing a better understanding of how implicit biases manifest and developing methods to interrupt these biases in educational work. This serves to help dance educators through the training, mentoring, and development of future dancers and dance educators. Policies and protocol become particularly poignant to consider in training programs, assessment models, and gatekeeping mechanisms within the field of dance and specifically in dance education. Certifying bodies, educational institutions, and member organizations must also attend to how language and institutional structures reify or disrupt the implicit biases found not just at the larger level through quantitative data tracking but also in the interpersonal exchanges at the micro-level of person-to-person interactions.

There are psychological aspects that are not only an element of the implicit bias itself, but also an element of how students, applicants, colleagues perceive selection processes, biases, and decisions. In research on the psychology of perceived discrimination, two models emerge. In one model, perceivers of discrimination adhere to a "**prototype model**," wherein players in the decision-making process are assumed to adhere to roles of the victim and perpetrator that align with the perceiver's understanding of those roles. This model calls upon dance applicants, for example, to think of the non-disabled, White head of the program as the perpetrator and the disabled person of color applicant as the victim based on their identity markers and roles in the process, no matter what careful deliberations and decision-making took place. In the prototype model, a dance applicant may assume the non-disabled, White head of the program was the reason a disabled person of color was not accepted, when it could have been some other reason entirely unrelated to these identity markers.

In the second model, the "organizational justice model," the structures in place in the decision-making process explicitly relay, "procedural, informational, interpersonal, and distributive fairness,"[7] The second model is about the explicit display, performance, and disclosure of the mechanisms that organize the decision-making process. In this **organizational justice model**, sharing with applicants how decisions are made is a way for administrators, evaluators, assessors, and other decision-making gatekeepers to make their process transparent. This proactively transparent explanation of the deliberation process can illuminate the level of attention the gatekeepers have put into disrupting bias. It also displays a willingness to involve the community in accountability measures for their decision-making protocols. The transparency of the decision-making process can both ensure accountability to anti-bias and equitable determinations, as well as display evidence of this attempt to comply with such goals to the applicants. This more thorough disclosure of the process reduces the feelings of distrust or lack of fairness in the applicant pool in effect heading off perceived inequity or unfairness before feelings of distrust can fester.

Disrupt Implicit Biases

We start to see good and bad news in the above discussion of how transparency can change the perceptions and feelings about an evaluation or selection process in dance education as well as uncover where the negative effects of bias occur in the process. As explained in the concepts of implicit memory and priming in the Introduction, the bad news is that the brain-body is susceptible to suggestion, and the good news is that the brain-body is susceptible to suggestion. As with the intentional transparency described above in the organizational justice model, there are rather small changes an educator can implement that changes the experiences and messages for students and applicants. Much of the reason we hold the biases we hold are due to the suggestions we receive via personal life experiences, what social science calls implicit memories, from media messages to family background, friends, or collegial groups. Research suggests that even the most deeply held biases can be altered in a number of often unnoticeable ways by introducing alternative messages to counter what a person has previously been exposed to. Fleeting suggestions to the brain to ignore its existing bias result in short-term effects that counter that bias. Over long periods of interrupting a bias, there is evidence that the interruptions have more lasting effects.[8] Based on this research, finding creative ways to *trick* the mind can have significant implications for disrupting bias. Over time, some of those *tricks* may even become immersive and transformative in daily interactions and relationships. Educational institutions are a great example of this. Over long periods of time, students are exposed to the assumptions and values present in their learning environments. These often alter a student's perspectives, interests, behaviors, practices, and even their culture within the school setting. We as educators create communities and environments that immerse students in the norms of the field of dance over their time studying with us that affect the way they understand and perceive the field of dance.

Tricking the Mind: Disrupting Implicit Biases

In a similar way that magicians or mentalists deliver suggestions to the subconscious mind that present to the conscious mind as magic, the mechanisms of implicit bias can also be disrupted, only this trick you may not notice.[9] The term in social science, as described in the Introduction, is *priming*. Malcolm Gladwell, in his book *Blink: The Power of Thinking Without Thinking*, provides an example of priming where test subjects walk down a hallway to a room where they engage in an activity of reordering a series of five-word combinations into sentences as quickly as possible.[10] After completing this task, the students then return back down the hallway, walking slower than they did when arriving to take the test. This is due to a series of words scattered within the word groups they arranged that brought about suggestions of old age, including words like "gray," "old," and "wrinkle." These words were placed as a primer to determine whether placing them with no attention to their thematic connection could affect the behavior of those who participated in the activity. With a bit of creativity, we as dance educators can positively influence students in similar subconscious ways.

In the dance world this might look something like making intentional choices, as mentioned in the Introduction, of what visual posters a teacher puts on the studio or classroom walls to suggest what types of dances are valued or included. Through intentional priming by establishing visual and curricular examples of a diverse array of atypical dancers, educators can disrupt assumptions about socially ubiquitous messages of White, thin, non-disabled-bodied, gender-conforming individuals representing what dancers look like. The more examples the mind takes in, the more implicit memories it has to aggregate, creating a fuller representation of what a dancer looks like. Even something as seemingly innocuous as a computer screensaver with positive, empowered images of marginalized groups of dancers and dance forms can have an effect on whether the mind can see atypical representations of dancers as normative.[11]

For example, if you have identified a stereotypical notion that is prevalent amongst students in a class or even in your own thinking, creating quizzes that provide examples that contradict that stereotype can have short-term effects on disrupting that particular area of bias. Take, for instance, the assumption that ballet is a universal foundation for all dance forms. Before having a conversation about the importance of ballet in a dance history class, an instructor may come up with a short quiz in which a student must determine where a dance form may have originated from based on a picture or short video clip of a dance form. In this quiz, the instructor may have only included dance forms that are unrelated to ballet or to Western dance forms in general. Even if the quiz does not directly relate to the area of focus for the class discussion, the mere exposure to the images affects the subconscious mind, thereby influencing what moves into consciousness when considering ideas and concepts in the class discussion. In short, the more exposure the mind has to experiences that run counter to the established bias, the more kindling it has to ignite a new perspective that runs counter to the previously established bias even if for a short term.

The longer one is exposed to messages and experiences that contradict the held belief or attitude, the longer lasting the effects of the disruption. Thinking about society, when dominant groups and marginalized groups come together in an environment that fosters equitable exchange and reveals the fallacious nature of stereotypes they may have held toward each other, biases do tend to be upended. Think about how public school desegregation challenged the minds of some and changed the minds of other White people who had never been in close proximity to Black students. The dominant group tends to have a diminished fervor for previously held negative beliefs about that marginalized or oppressed group. But beware, and take caution. Eberhardt's work informs us that the same may not take place for marginalized members of a community, because in the process of the dominant group unlearning their stereotypes and transforming the negative attitudes they once held about the marginalized group to positive attitudes, there can be a considerable amount of microaggressions discovered by the marginalized group of just what the dominant group thinks of them.[12]

Eberhardt also reminds her reader of Allport's[13] research identifying that all cross-cultural interaction does not reduce implicit bias. Some environments increase implicit bias. In environments where dominant and marginalized groups encounter anxiety-inducing or competition-based, short and infrequent amounts of time with each other, these exchanges will more likely exacerbate implicit biases. This is why the environments created in a studio or classroom must be intentional if they are to reduce implicit bias among students, between instructors, and in the relationship between students and instructors. Stated succinctly, community matters and should be intentionally scrutinized with an eye toward disrupting the negative effects of implicit biases.

A strategy to continue the personal and collective work of disrupting the influence of implicit bias is to intentionally and actively include and seek out the expertise of historically marginalized dancers and educators, or those with different affinities for movement than you have that can offer a counterpoint to your observational sensibilities. If there are no members of these groups whom you are close to or you find you respect, take a breath.

The efficacy of systemic oppression is working the way it is intended to by maintaining divisions between groups of people, silencing and dismissing some while celebrating and comforting others. There may be deeper preliminary work that needs to be done to examine the ways your life has not brought you in close proximity to dancers, educators, or dance educators who are members of historically marginalized groups. You must now disrupt those structures in order to begin forging those relationships.

To illustrate the value of these connections, I share this lived experience. I was with a group of visual and performing artists at the Guggenheim Museum. When the group began to share its experiences when viewing Picasso's *Woman Ironing*, one group of observers shared that the woman looked healthy. Another group shared strong objections to this analysis. In a discussion that ensued, both groups pointed to the yellow hues and the thin frame of the woman as evidence to support their position. While both groups were pulling from the same objective aspects of the painting, one group interpreted the yellow-hued, thin woman as glowing and healthy, while the other group interpreted her hue and thin frame to be markers of jaundice and malnutrition. Of particular intrigue to me was that the observers who perceived the woman to be healthy were White-bodied artists, while those who perceived the woman as unhealthy were Black-bodied artists.

If such different interpretations of the same objective aspects of an artwork take place even in observing a still image, imagine the complexities at play in the analysis of the ever-changing moving body. Even with the argument that within the ephemeral nature of our moving content, there are repeated patterns that arise from the movement, because we are dynamic creatures of habit. Who determines what patterns are attributed to the student moving and what patterns are created based on prior experiences in the minds of the dance educator? Who can determine whether or not the patterns that arise for the educator are subconsciously predetermined by some stimulus that is not actually present in the sociocultural environment in which the student is moving? A deeper understanding of how observation and analysis work is critical to understanding what is taking place when these implicit biases are exacerbated in dance education.

Immersion: Long-Term Solutions for Interrupting Biases

This brings us back to the work of Moore and Yamamoto mentioned in earlier chapters. Here, I focus on the authors' discussion of how body prejudice in connection to upending implicit biases in a more sustained, long-term practice, can result in long-term shifts in implicit biases.[14] In relation to movement observation, there are a few key elements that affect the accuracy of analysis and evaluation and intersect with the research on implicit bias in dance education. One component is the necessity to expand the movement experiences across cultures in the studio and classroom. Moore and Yamamoto include in the list of determinants that affect accuracy of observation and analysis "the similarity of cultural and social backgrounds between the mover and observer, their personal familiarity with each other, as well as their motivations and needs to understand one another."[15] I posit that this consideration is relative and is dependent on the individual context and perceptions of those students and educators involved.

The level of similarity between student and educator backgrounds is based on the frame a person has access to or choses to orient the comparison. For example, in comparing Appalachian clogging and South African gumboot dancing, one person could frame their comparison around racial differences in the cultures, while another person could frame their comparison around percussiveness of the dance forms? If so, they will perceive the comparisons differently using these different frames of reference. In a classroom, if a teacher has not shared much of their background, hobbies, or other ways to connect with their students, the students have little in the way of options to frame how they are similar in background and thus can relate to their teacher.

The relationship is also dependent on how ingrained either person is in relevant aspects of Social Dominance Orientation (SDO) discussed in earlier chapters. Are there established notions of group superiority present in how students and educators are perceiving each other? How steeped are the students and educators in notions that there are some people that are better than others based on aspects of their identity or genre of dance they study? If this is a significant factor for a student or educator, it may be more challenging to perceive the similarities between their cultures if aspects of supremacy of one group over another underlie perceptions about each other. What aspects of similarity are the focus for the student and educator? For example, are dance educators focusing more on aspects of energy or Effort while students are organizing their movement around aspects of cardinal direction orientation of facings? Is there a way that students and educators can better align and understand what their areas of focus are with regard to similarity of movement? These are the questions that need to be asked and discussed in order to break open the assumptions that underlie understanding each other. I also posit that with fully invested curiosity and deep listening to each other, devoid of notions of superiority, familiarity between individuals can be cultivated and result in deeper understanding between students and educators. Of course, this is a very personal and discrete experience that takes time to foster.

Research on the influences of implicit bias in daily life now shows that some of the most superficial and perfunctory interactions between people can expand the familiarity between individuals when the exposure between those people runs counter to the existing stereotypes people have about each other. Exposure that is taken in even through passive exposure, such as a computer screensaver, can shift ingrained stereotypes and biases. Moore and Yamamoto assert that expanding private lexicons and experiences with cultures and groups a person is unfamiliar with can enhance the accuracy of movement analysis. This assertion is supported by the work of social science research on how implicit biases can be reduced by this exposure to counter-stereotypes.[16] I assert that the same can be said of movement evaluation and interpretation in dance classes. The more that both educators and students understand and have a familiarity with each other's cultural reference points, the more accurate and empathetic those cross-cultural interpretations can be, thus disrupting the divisive hold of implicit biases.

To continue this growth and process of inhibiting the negative influences of implicit biases means we need to continue to have close connection, discussion, and culturally responsive engagement with each other as a community of consummate dance learners and educators. We should do this not only within dance education communities but also across other fields of learning. Having conversations with people who are out-group members to the field of dance and dance education can bring much needed new questions and curiosities.

Finding Common Ground: The Benefit of Naming Implicit Biases

An example of the value of this exchange came when I was having a discussion with a colleague at my institution. She conducts education research on implicit bias in faculty hiring processes. When I explained to her that I was examining the effects of implicit bias in dance education, she responded with a bit of perplexed curiosity. I then asked if she could say more about what was perplexing about the idea of implicit bias in dance education. She shared that, while there was ample research about the manifestations of implicit bias in the STEM fields because of the importance of empirical, unbiased distance in research processes in STEM fields, she was unclear what the benefits of examining implicit bias in the arts would garner if the arts were not about being unbiased.

I realized in her inquiry that there were insider cultural assumptions I had made about the intersections of bias and dance that needed to be articulated explicitly. While the notion of objectivity and the importance of repeatable testing or research procedures are hallmarks of STEM fields, this is not the case in the arts. It is as important for me to articulate how differently I approach my creative sensibilities as it is important for audiences to display some sort of felt sense or bias when encountering the work. I assert that the study, discovery, or "outing" of implicit biases should be addressed or handled in the subjective, creative, personal, lived experience areas of creative research. This is the value in examining the role implicit biases play in the arts that occurs simultaneously with the negative effects implicit biases can bring into educational and selection processes in dance environments.

First, as a teacher aligned with the realization that objectivity is a myth and that personal and cultural factors color so much of how people see the world, I do not suggest that implicit bias study in dance education should be about producing formulaic, repeatable, non-creative processes as empirical areas of study. I believe that the field of dance and more specifically dance education should continue to think critically about the needs of their students and make thoughtful adjustments as the creative, improvisational educators in the field of dance often do. The discovery of implicit biases in each individual should be used to do two things: (1) modify an individual's personal creative processes to disrupt the negative effects of implicit bias on collaborators and students and (2) reveal and unveil for each person a deeper understanding of themselves and each other as it relates to their personal biases and the lived experiences that seed their own creative work, processes, and sensibilities. Examining why we hold certain preferences provides a valuable opportunity to better see ourselves as artists and as educators. It also provides the opportunity to share a clearer picture of ourselves with others through our creative work. An added benefit is becoming more aware of the ways that implicit biases are in conflict with conscious biases and aesthetic preferences. This discovery has the potential to more clearly hone creative work into the aesthetic landscape dancers, artists, and educators intend to create and relay.

As the discussion that ensued in the *Woman Ironing* story I shared earlier in this chapter illuminates, the value of seeing each other more clearly as creative individuals through uniquely refined and articulated personal experiences and perspectives could lead to deeper human connection to each other. These deeper connections would honor and celebrate differences in taste as sites to negotiate vulnerable human connection and understanding between people. Had the implicit biases carried by each faction of the discussion about the Picasso painting not been addressed, the potential for disagreement, frustration, and further assumptions about each other would have been rife. In that example, each group instead could clearly delineate that it has very different associations with thin bodies and with the color yellow when presented as a hue on a human body.

A next step for this group of artists could be to continue the discussion after self-reflection or a search through personal experiences to track where these messages about the color yellow were created, or to discuss the social structures that resulted in these assumptions and how one version operates as dominant in society. This process carries in it the burgeoning possibility for developing a common ground of understanding each other's perspective, not uniformity or dominance of one perspective over another. It has the potential to move individuals and communities beyond a right-wrong paradigm or unified standard perspective as the condition for connection and instead offer a paradigm of empathic understanding of different perspectives as the condition for connection.

Naming and exploring explicit biases while discovering and unpacking implicit biases can create understanding about how societal messages affect meaning-making in teaching, creative processes, and collaborative work, as well as in daily exchanges. This practice of deep questioning and internal investigation, coupled with connection to community has the capacity to move educators and artists toward honoring the subjective reality of difference in human experiences and associations. With a conscious disposition toward more equitable representation of genres and aesthetics, coupled with addressing the centering of dominant perspectives while marginalizing others, there is also the potential to move the field of dance education toward a more equitable and inclusive environment. In various aspects of life, examining how implicit and explicit biases are in operation can assist with a goal of generating and understanding multiple ideas and perspectives, rather than expecting one group to conform to one idea or another.

The Predicament of Complicity

This process of interpersonal connection and deep listening takes great care and adaptability for every community, as each member is unique in some ways and part of a larger social system of power in other ways. Each environment is wholly unique in unanticipated ways that must be considered. For example, are you asking marginalized members of your dance community to be complicit in the hegemonic messages that continue to perpetuate their oppression? Accountability and sensitivity to the positions you place marginalized or disenfranchised people in, especially students for whom you are holding their grades, certifications, credentialing, references, and by extension, their futures in your hands, is important. Epistemic injustice research indicates that the person in the room with the most social power is often the person who gets to set the tone, truths, and assumptions in the room, unchallenged by those with a different set of sentiments on the context, situation, or circumstances.[17] The privilege of testimonial injustice, described in Chapter 4 lies with the person in the room with the most social power, i.e., in the context of the classroom or educational program teachers and students of a privileged in-group.

It is likely that marginalized community members, including students and colleagues, have experienced the negative effects of speaking a different *truth* or set of experiences, values, or knowledges. For the purposes of self-preservation, it is unlikely that a student or colleague who is either an underrepresented member of the community or a historically marginalized member of society will challenge the biases, assumptions, or ways in which those historically dominant or in-group members *have it wrong* from their perspective. For some marginalized group members, they have determined from their lived experiences that their success in life depends on indoctrination into these dominant systems of knowledge. They may have experienced upset when the promise of success either came with too much of a loss of a sense of self and culture or an inability to ever really fit in and succeed on equal terms with their dominant-group counterparts no matter their level of conformity.

Instead of hiding behind the realities of being in a dominant group or position of power, as we all have been at one time or another in lives, seek out opportunities to use the privileges that come with that in-group status to support those out-group members. Particularly in the U.S. where robust performative attention-getting displays making demands and voicing opinions can so often be linked with dominant social group status, if there is an urge to show support through an emphatic performance of outrage, encouragement, or care, you may be doing it wrong. This is actually a behavioral manifestation of a pattern of privilege to perform your thoughts and feelings unapologetically, to claim space of dominant status in a room. As Sara Ahmed so eloquently reminds us in relation to racism, the mere naming or calling out of inequity does not *do* a thing, but is rather a performance of a thing.[18] To disrupt inequity takes ongoing action, accountability, vulnerability to get it wrong from time to time, and an empathy for and collaboration with others.

Instead of boisterously calling out injustice with little regard to the effects of your assertion potentially further stigmatizing out-group members, I suggest checking in with out-group members privately to first acknowledge you felt a sense of exclusionary behavior or inequity and ask how they felt about it. There are instances where publicly attesting that you have identified an inequity is actually more damaging to the professional well-being and social sense of belonging of the marginalized group member. The social stigma afforded the marginalized person may increase if they are put at the center of conversation in a way that places them in the vulnerable position of the object of resentments of dominant group members uncomfortable with this challenge to their power and privilege.

After speaking with the marginalized person or people you feel were or could be harmed, if there is a comfort level and trust developed over time between you and the out-group member, you may ask how you can be of support in future instances of inequity. These interpersonal connections with marginalized group members may take time to foster when they are not guided solely by power dynamics and instead by personal connection. Trust and open communication is something that is earned, not an entitlement, nor is it fostered simply by reading books and understanding the concepts that undergird inequity and oppression. An ongoing reflective and embodied practice of listening and developing new embodied practices that disrupt habits of dominant social behavior is incumbent in developing human connection across power dynamics.

A Somatic Approach/Attuning/Check-In

As a moment of connection to this notion of ongoing reflective embodied practice and also a recuperation from structures, systems, and quantitative, objective approaches, I ask that you remember the sensate body and the power and knowledge systems located in embodied inquiry. Remember that the world of implicit biases are that of habitual patterns thrust on people by societal mechanisms. These are patterns that we have lived in for so long that we cannot see or differentiate them or reimagine through any other frames of reference without intentional study and practice. I ask that you now consider the methodologies of somatic practices as a disrupter to the cognitive dissonance that results from undoing implicit biases. When asking reflective questions about your own personal biases and that of your organization, do not forget to track the sensations of how your body is feeling as you explore. If it is possible to concede to two premises: (1) biases are based on habits and (2) slowing down to track their presence and manifestation in the body can result in new ways of practicing and moving in the world, I argue that emergent, mind-body approaches have the potential or capacity to undo some of the harm of living blindly into the negative influences of biases.

Self-reflective questioning that examines the foundations of both existing explicit biases and discovered implicit biases can help in the process of sitting with and reflecting upon the nature of those biases and how they may have unintended consequences in your daily attitudes, decisions, and behaviors. The crucial aspect that somatics offers to this self-reflection is the importance of tracking or centering internal, felt sensations when interacting with sociopolitical systems of power, privilege, and oppression. This is essential no matter whether you stand as a dominant group member or marginalized group member in any context or relationship to the power dynamic. This process does not fly in opposition to the call of social somatics to engage in a relational exploration of the body in community.[19] Rather, it asks that people track the momentary, fleeting sensations, thoughts, feelings of entitlement or discomfort, hurt or dehumanization in interactions with others as it relates to socially constructed biases.

The first step in this somatic process is the practice of slowing down the patterning, whether that be of thought, language, or behavior, and tracking the sensations in the body as cognitive dissonance arises. Becoming familiar with the sensations that show up in the body in moments of cognitive dissonance may help in more quickly recognizing those sensations and identifying cognitive dissonance in the future. Take the time to examine and reorient to this change in self-perception, and grapple with aspects of identity. The disconnect between how you may see yourself and how this discovery may misalign with the effects that biases are having on your relationship with others and the environment may take some time to process or sort through. In slowing down and working through a self-reflexive process, it is important to track defense mechanisms that may explain away discoveries about bias. This is a great opportunity to engage with accountability partners around this discovery. These are people who are knowledgeable about the structural, behavioral, and interpersonal inequities seeded by the particular area of biases discovered. More about finding and working in community with others will come later in Chapter 6.

Even in considering the value of somatic practices in undoing negative effects of some of the implicit and explicit biases, the field of somatics also holds cultural biases within it. When I take a step back to examine the larger concept of reintegration of mind and body, which is central to somatics, I acknowledge that the disconnect between mind and body stems from the disruptive effects of the Cartesian split born in the Western world within the cultural context of Western colonization around the globe. There were cultures, societies, and world views that predate this Cartesian duality that did not move through the world adhering to this body-mind chasm. If the concept of somatics is to re-integrate the body to resolve the embodied losses resulting from thinking of the mind and body as separate in the Western understandings of existence, this means there are potential systems of knowledge that either maintain remnants of a wholly integrated body-mind consciousness or that had minimal or negligent loss of this fully integrated sense of themselves and the world. From Haiti to Japan, many of the somatic movement practices that exist today have pulled from cultures and peoples who did not submit to a sense of the mind and body being separate or to the body being subordinate in value to the mind.[20]

This is another moment in which to slow down language, understanding, and practices and interrogate the idea that the concept of somatics is one of the Western World. This is only true in the way that Christopher Columbus discovered an already existing continent of people. I mention this as another example in the field of dance and dance education that the privilege of predominantly White, Western-centered value systems can cloud a fuller understanding of a plethora of ways to check in with the body-mind and assess how inner sentiments, sensations, and patterns show up in dance studios and classrooms. There are practices from the swaying, humming, and praise dances of Black churches to chanting, breathing, and shared meals of Buddhist sanghas that offer non–Western somatic practices developed by people of color. Another offering from this line of thought is an invitation to upend the notion that somatic practices exist only in predominantly White spaces and cultures. There are somatic practices that are both created by non–Western BIPOC cultures and are practiced in BIPOC communities.

To disrupt this notion of somatics being a concept of a White, Western world of practitioners, seek out further examination of what somatic practices can be a site of learning, processing, and repatterning. A place to begin this search is exploring the work of scholars like Don Hanlon Johnson in his book *Diverse Bodies, Diverse Practices: Toward an Inclusive Somatics*.[21] This book explores BIPOC voices discussing connections between the field of somatics and practices specific to their identities and cultural backgrounds. For further investigation, seek out opportunities to forge genuine relationships with BIPOC somatic practitioners as colleagues or as clients in their modalities.

Sustained relationships and community-building deepens the immersion into these somatic systems and approaches to viewing the moving body, systems of knowledge, and the world around us. One example I can name is the full year of somatic practice and culture-building in a diverse community of people through Karine Bell's Rooted Global Village organization.[22] With a clear intention of exploring and checking implicit biases' negative effects, these relationships can promote the disruption of biased assumptions about the expertise of stigmatized practitioners. Key to this process is attuning to the body when the discomfort and dissonance of implicit bias emerges. This attuning is a powerful practice in disrupting the negative effects of implicit bias.

6

Numbers, Qualities, and Bodies

Solutions for Implicit Bias

Thus far in the book, I have discussed manifestations, feeders, and disruptors of implicit bias in the context of dance education. Now I turn to what solutions there are to combat the negative effects of implicit bias in the dance studio and classroom settings. Is it even possible to counter the effects of implicit biases that are, by definition, unable to be perceived by the conscious mind? Holroyd asserts that even before research on implicit bias was conducted, people were capable of realizing when there was a behavior or belief that did not align with the person's conscious beliefs or internal logic.[1] Banaji and Greenwald call these moments "blind spots."[2] In Holroyd's work, she argues, "insofar as these observations are blocked by motivated ignorance—avoidance or ignoring (perhaps subconsciously) of evidence that serves one's goals—or self-deception, or excessive weight given to misleading introspective evidence, a failure to have this sort of awareness is culpable to some degree."[3] Now with more extensive research on the negative effects of implicit bias, its manifestations, and disruptors, Holroyd asserts that once you are aware of the bias, you are certainly responsible for efforts to disrupt its negative effects moving forward.

A tested and relatively accessible way to learn more about your implicit biases comes in the form of the Implicit Association Test (IAT) mentioned earlier in the book. The Harvard University's Project Implicit website[4] guides the participant through a series of potential points of bias from racial biases to weight bias to disability bias and more. The tests ask that you look at a series of images and select a certain category of words while looking at the image. For example, selecting words you might consider positive while looking at various images of White or Black people. The amount of time it takes the participant to select the word, or the accuracy of selecting the appropriate word, determines the level of bias.

There are a number of ways that social scientists and empirical psychologists who are studying how the mind is affected by implicit biases use quantitative research in highly controlled experiments to determine its effects. Creatively integrating evidence-based solutions in our classrooms is a practical and creative endeavor best addressed by educators in their respective settings. The general research findings coupled with the specifics of each of our diverse teaching settings and our particular care and expertise in performative, embodied, and reflective practices are most efficacious for addressing the issues of implicit bias. For this reason, I have organized a discussion of solutions, many examples of which are found throughout the book, into the categories of quantitative or data-tracking measures; qualitative or interpersonal, sociocultural, contextual measures; and embodied practices and attuned behavioral measures. I do not, however, treat proposed solutions as definitive, formulaic solutions to be replicated without full consideration of the circumstances and specific context of your educational setting. There must be a level of nuance in how we combat implicit bias, and this high level of critical thinking should be integral to implementing any solutions proposed in this chapter in your own educational setting.

Quantitative Solutions

Keeping track of demographic data that enables an educator or administrator to see in numerical, evidentiary ways how biases are affecting behavior is a quantitative solution that disrupts the negative effects of implicit bias. This mode of disruption is best used when tracking grading or recorded assessment, deliberations and selection processes, or simple behavioral markers that do not include dense, detailed information to track—tracking which students are called on in each class session described in Chapter 5, for example. These measures are about seeing the numbers and percentages involved in different aspects of decision making and behaviors over time.

An example of this type of quantitative tracking comes from the scholarship selection process I was involved in implementing, where the applicant pool was compared to both the demographics of the organization's membership broadly and to the smaller applicant pool for the scholarship. To ensure the percentages either remained consistent throughout each step of the selection process or favored historically marginalized and underrepresented groups, demographic information about race, gender identity, sexual preference, and socioeconomic status were kept throughout the process. This data was hidden during the deliberation process and then made visible to the selection committee, in numerical format separate from the applications themselves, after their selections had been made. At that point in the deliberation, the selection committee could see in the data whether they had maintained the demographic ratios of the original applicant pool at each stage of deliberation without knowledge of identities of the applicant while reviewing the applications. This example makes clear that these data-tracking measures can be descriptive, illuminating what has taken place thus far in the process. They can also be prescriptive accountability measures that ensure equity is maintained based on the established standard set moving forward in the selection process. In this case, the standard was to maintain the demographic percentages of those who applied. In the future, this standard could be more in line with the restorative justice model of equity and move to a standard of maintaining demographic percentages that are twice the percentage of historically marginalized applicants being accepted, for example. In this version of the selection process, the selection committee would rank each blinded application. Then have only the demographic information associated with each corresponding application number revealed to select the top applicants from each demographic category. The organization could also decide to maintain the demographic representation of their full membership in the selection process if they chose to do so.

Upon reviewing demographic benchmarks, educators or administrators may realize the pool of applicant options is not sufficient in order to meet these demographic accountability measures. There may be some cognitive dissonance that develops in which people begin to share reasons why there is little recourse to adhere to the benchmarks based on the applicant pool. In a 2015 speech, Dr. Banaji, co-author of the book *Blindspot: Hidden Biases of Good People*, shared a story regarding the goal of hiring women into a higher education faculty position.[5] When the hiring process in her program did not produce an applicant pool that statistically mirrored the percentage of women in the field in which they were hiring, her search committee suspended the search and contacted top experts in the field to make recommendations of people who would be well-qualified for the position with no mention of the gender disparity in the original search. That inquiry resulted in a number of highly-qualified potential women applicants. These women were contacted and invited to apply.

After completing their interview, they were asked why they did not initially apply for the position. A number of the women responded that they did not feel qualified or feel like appropriate candidates for the position. This was a function of self-directed stigma and internalized

6. Numbers, Qualities, and Bodies 139

oppression, described in Chapter 1, wherein the stigmatized person maintains the very bias that negatively affects them. Also functioning in this example are the effects of cultural cloning, where a person assumes they don't meet the established identity markers for the people most commonly represented in that position. These inclinations are common to marginalized out-group communities and should be considered in the application processes educational programs design.

There are two things to note in this example of a hiring process. The first is that the selection committee halted the selection process when the applicant pool did not meet the established benchmarks of demographic representation. The hiring committee then designed a more targeted and directed process that sought out talent rather than asking talent to seek out the position. Second, there was evidence of the marginalized group exhibiting remnants of internalized oppression in which they had determined themselves to be less qualified, worthy, or likely to be considered for the position. If an organization is committed to the established goals of equity, it is vital to disrupt mechanisms that do not produce the intended goals articulated in the selection process. If the selection process does not result in the intended pool of applicants, the onus is on the program to correct for bias, because it bears a more significant role through its privileges and access to power in disrupting systemic inequities and resulting biases. Shifting responsibility onto prospective applicants does not address an ineffective recruitment model and/or application process that does not meet the established goals for equitable representation.

Now back to the example of how to establish accountability in a selection process that comes from my work in advising a dance organization. Within the confines and culture of this organization, I advised on how it could establish quantitative measures to track equitable representation. At the time I began working with the organization, it was seeking to establish an accountability strategy to monitor, ensure, and increase representation of marginalized members of the organization as it related specifically to race, LGBTQ, and regional representation in the selection process for membership, awards, and scholarships. First, the organization began tracking demographic information on all members. For every membership renewal and any other application process, demographic information was taken about race, sexuality and gender identity, regional location, population density it served, and income or socioeconomic class information.

After aggregating that data, it was then able to track what the actual percentages were of underrepresented groups both in the applicant pool itself and in comparison to the entire membership pool. The organization then had staff members, who did not deliberate about the applications, remove the demographic information from the materials provided to application reviewers. After the initial rubric-based blind review and ranking of applications, the selection committee then looked at the anonymous demographic statistics of the applicants via application numbers. It then selected the top-ranking applicants that met the demographic percentages of the applicant pool.

What was most encouraging and brought pride to the evaluators is that the process was such that there were many applicants from marginalized populations to choose from in the top tier of the criteria selection. It was not a struggle to ensure that the demographic representation percentages were met. Not only was the organization able to determine that its own personal, evaluative sensibilities did not promote discrimination against marginalized members of the applicant pool in the review process, it now had data and a clear and transparent protocol of how selections were made for accountability that it could proudly share evidence of with members. The transparency of sharing the process with member of the organization and more specifically to the applicant pool of how the process is designed to disrupt implicit bias shifted the perception of discrimination from the prototype model to the organizational justice model both described in Chapter 5.

This level of numerical tracking of marginalized groups in a community and how they are supported or alienated in the evaluation process is a useful tool in helping an organization understand what, via evidence and transparency, is happening in the selection processes of the organization. This sort of numerical tracking not only helps evidence an organization or program's commitment to accountability, but it can also illuminate where any potential challenges to equitable representation show up in the process. Identification of where challenges of equity show up in the process can then be addressed in policies, protocols, and procedural changes in future decision-making processes.

Policy, Procedure, and Decision-Making

Accountability measures are a way to assess whether the institution or classroom teacher is doing what they claim to be doing and are doing so in an equitable manner. Policies and procedures are a place to ensure consistency and fairness for all students and colleagues. Those policies and procedures that are organized to prevent the effects of implicit bias must be applied consistently across the board in order for them to truly be equitable. Each exception is either the result of a policy or procedure that is not written well enough to apply to everyone, or is the evidence of implicit bias creating a mind bug[6] of why there should be an exception for this one

6. Numbers, Qualities, and Bodies   141

case that ultimately reifies the implicit bias. When events come up wherein exceptions to a rule or procedure seem warranted, I recommend taking time to do an examination of the errant policy. If the policy is not effectively working for every person, it needs to be examined and amended to ensure that it can and does apply equitably to everyone.

For example, in the above-mentioned case of my work with the dance organization in its scholarship selection process, the organization had lost the trust of members of the organization who represent historically marginalized populations in the U.S., including the BIPOC and LGBTQ communities. The protocol I proposed instituted a numerical rubric that identified a demographic baseline of who applied for the scholarship, then tracked whether the demographic ratio was maintained for the entire selection process. For example, if 40 percent of the applicant pool selected the racial identifier of Black, I proposed to track whether that percentage remained consistent across each level of the selection process. Not only did a consistent percentage of demographic ratios throughout the process bear out, but participants in this process advocated for applicants who extended beyond the required minimums for the historically marginalized groups in the organization.

This shifted the organization from the now rather commonplace equity model of inclusion into a more radical, restorative justice approach. In the restorative justice model, the goal is not simply to maintain equity in the present, but, rather, to repair the damage or resulting harm caused by historical injustices. This model calls on gatekeepers to consider not just what equity looks like in the current demographic landscape, but also ask what equity would look like today had there not been historical, systemic injustices that result in the demographic dynamics that we have today.

There are two ways to use this demographic accountability protocol. One is to track and glean how the numbers bear out in each stage of the selection process. This way of using demographic tracking helps members of the selection process see how the process is or is not affected by implicit biases that eliminate historically marginalized populations from the pool. Through numerical representation, it tracks how the demographic percentages may wax or wane throughout the selection process.

The second way to use this demographic accountability process is a more proactive application. The deciding body can set a goal or benchmark of what percentages for the various population representations they would like to meet. For example, the goal may simply be to maintain the demographic percentages of applicants. In communities committed to a more restorative justice approach, the goal or benchmark may be to select twice the number of historically marginalized or underrepresented people who applied, who are among the membership, or who are in the U.S. in their selection process. What is important is that the structure of the numerical tracking helps the selection committee maintain a diligent, measurable structure for determining how well they are meeting the goals they have committed to. This process helps keep track of how successful they are at rooting out the negative effects of implicit bias and how to make changes to better meet their goals of equity and inclusion.

In order to account for underrepresented people in these processes, it is beneficial to maintain quantitative goals and tracking procedures wherein the faculty-administrators are able to ensure that the demographics of marginalized student/faculty needs are met while also still upholding the selection rubrics, standards, and criteria in a way that apply to all applicants. When a policy is no longer working for everyone, especially when it is not working for historically marginalized groups, it should be corrected, amended, improved upon until it does. It should not be kept only to carve out exceptions on a case-by-case basis. Exceptions are the byproduct of implicit decision-making that was not communicated explicitly to those who applied. If there are exceptions, it is advantageous to equity goals that attempts to be explicit are made for all stakeholders. And yes, this is a challenging and at times radical task in the existing structures of education. Accountability and transparency are necessary aspects for radical change that moves toward a more inclusive and equitable learning community.

Another method from the world of empiricism is to create a level of objective or equal replication in relating to students. It is imperative to balance the need for unique and personal connections to each student with what I call the emotional detachment of the educator's relationship with students. I have been there myself, experiencing the tugging at my heart strings of a personal situation with a student that beckons me to make an exception just this once. While having personal relationships with students is certainly a benefit to the teacher-student relationship, it is imperative that stated behavioral consequences and performance assessments of students be met with a level of detachment wherein the teacher separates their personal sentiments from the actual work produced by the students. The instructor must separate the daily personal communication and exchange with students from the objective measures of student performance. Assessment, evaluation, and consequences should be determined outside of an educator's personal preference for or aversion to a student's personality.

This requires educators to take a breath or wait a day to settle the internal triggers a student may have set off before making decisions about the student's actual performance in the class. Educators must be able to assess each student on a consistent, equitable level of determinants that applies to every student. While this may seem simple, foundational, and rather apparent to many educators, it is important to remember that this is the conscious brain steeped in these sentiments of equity. Many of these momentary decisions and behaviors are influenced by the unconscious mechanisms of the brain, unbeknownst to the holder of the implicit bias.

In the larger classes I teach, I anonymize the writing assignments students turn in as a way to remove the negative effects of any implicit biases I may have for students in the class. When I have a class with large enrollment numbers that involves writing assignments throughout the course, I have implemented assigning each student a number the student uses in place of their name. The assigned number remains the same for the entire course in order to anonymously track the implementation of my suggestions throughout the duration of the course. This way, as I read the papers, I reduce the likelihood I am making assumptions about a student's name, an interaction we may have had, or something I witnessed during class. I am also still able to track any changes in a student's writing progress over the length of the course. This is an actionable tactic to disrupt implicit biases by reducing the effects of personal biases I may carry as an instructor. Of course, you may come to know and be very familiar with who the student may be based on what content they include in the writing assignment, or, of course, through any one-on-one meetings with a student about the content they are writing about, or to clarify your feedback on an assignment. But again, as a tactic for larger classes, you may also implement rotating grading duties with co-teachers, colleagues, or teaching assistants so that different people are grading different students each time a writing assignment is graded.

Quantitative tracking methods and empirical grading strategies such as the one described above can serve as a check on the dynamics of personal triggers, inclinations, and implicit biases. These methods also demonstrate ways of addressing the psychological phenomenon of implicit bias beyond objective measure. Instituting quantitative tracking in a class can also serve as a priming measure that addresses the aforementioned tactic of "tricking the mind." When there is an awareness that accountability is being tracked, the brain may hold in its consciousness the intention to be equitable in a way that, without the tracking, the effort slips into murky, unclear, or unconscious habits and patterns in the process that promote unwanted biases. Knowing that accountability and evidenced data is being collected brings into a crisper more formalized role the challenges and successes of inclusion and equity. The second phenomenon it addresses is the transparency of policies and protocols for students to reduce any perception of inequity as described in the organizational justice model in Chapter 5. These two phenomena point to the next area of focus on how to disrupt implicit bias that has to do more with the interpersonal and societal dynamics of the community.

Qualitative Solutions

Qualitative solutions to disrupting the negative effects of implicit bias are based on contextual factors of insider-outsider cultural dynamics, an understanding of historically marginalized societal disenfranchisement, and qualitative understandings of stigmatized group members, rather than on tracking quantifiable data. These methods of minimizing the effects of implicit bias are about a person's orientation and intentional attention to minimizing the effects of implicit bias in qualitative, socially contextual ways rather than numerical measurement or purported empirical processes. The extensive work in culturally relevant teaching and critical dance pedagogy that Dr. McCarthy-Brown has detailed in her book, *Dance Pedagogy for a Diverse World: Culturally Relevant Teaching in Theory, Research and Practice*, is a quick example of a qualitative solution model that is a detractor to in-group favoritism and implicit bias.[7] Teaching in a way that considers the larger systemic inequities of the U.S. society for your students and including resources and examples for students who are historically underrepresented or stigmatized in dance education are ways Dr. McCarthy-Brown details that can also disrupt implicit biases toward students in classes and intervene in the implicit biases students may carry for each other or for certain dance forms.

Once an implicit bias shifts into conscious awareness, there are a number of approaches a dance educator could enact to either disrupt or offset this bias of favoritism or aversion for students in a class. After realizing the implicit bias exists, some people may opt to decline to move forward with any preferential or discriminatory treatment they unearth, while others may choose to ensure that they incorporate additional underrepresented individuals in moments of additional attention or rewards in order to be more inclusive and advantageous toward those who are not included in the in-group favoritism. What tactic to take at any given point is a complex decision to make with numerous interconnecting dynamics of identity, culture, timing, and many other factors.

Objectivity and privileging numerical data do not always serve as the most effective solution to disrupt bias. There are circumstances in which the consideration of cultural, sociopolitical, or interpersonal dynamics are a potent resource to even asking the most effective empirical questions. Take Choreometrics, for example. Choreometrics is an area of study developed by ethnomusicologist Alan Lomax that considers dances across cultures in the field of dance ethnography. Choreometrics attempts to orient the study of movement to quantitative data. In so doing, however, it may miss contextual information. That contextual information includes the assumptions, biases, and personal experiences that affect the dance researcher's approach to establishing patterns, meaning, and connections to cultural contexts.

The process of grouping recurring patterns and constellations in Choreometrics is a wonderful example of the brain's ability to distill massive amounts of data into smaller abstracted categories. This process has as much to do with the categories we already have in place subconsciously as it does with the movement being observed. In the instance of Choreometrics, Bartenieff and Paulay[8] used elements focusing on Laban concepts of Effort and Shape to notate and organize massive amounts of data about human movement. When Effort and Shape are not central principles within the movement being observed, how does a researcher know they are asking the *right* questions to ascertain knowledge about the culture being studied?

Channeling Your Inner Ethnographer: A Case for the Value of Cultural Difference

Pulling from my own cross-cultural educational experiences and work in cross-cultural interactions and research methods, concepts from the field of dance ethnography are a significant way to deter the negative effects of implicit bias in my classroom. A cause for concern in disrupting implicit bias comes up in the idea proposed by Moore and Yamamoto with regard to accuracy of the analysis. They propose that movers and observers be of similar backgrounds and/or have a personal familiarity with one another in order to reduce divergent analysis of movement. While this assertion does seem rather logical, when I frame it in the context of cultural in-group and out-group dynamics and historical marginalization in teaching, this has the potential to exclude cultural outsiders of dominant cultural standards and frameworks, including colleagues and students, from engaging in opportunities that demonstrate their analytical proficiency.

Not only do such assertions exclude students and educators perceived to be of dissimilar backgrounds or without a personal connection to one another from being selected as resources for learning, it stunts the observations by reifying assumptions often shared when observer(s) and mover(s) are of a similar dominant culture background and/or maintain a relationship. Observers who have a discerning eye or ability to synthesize movement experiences into evocative description and analysis, but who have no connection to the mover or movement style of the in-group or dominant culture can benefit the observation process by offering new ways of seeing, perceiving, and inquiring about movement. This learning opportunity in cross-cultural observer-mover interactions is applicable in dance studios and classrooms. It also requires those with an expertise in the dance form being observed to articulate their perspectives in an explicit way to the observer from a different cultural background so that there is an equitable exchange of knowledge, rather than a fixed, definitive perspective.

I had a high school dance class that was a diverse mix of students from the African and Asian diasporas, Latinx students, and White students. The significant number of White students with competition dance training from local studios would choreograph evocative phrases that included splits and fan rolls. I encouraged two Latina students to choreograph a Bachata dance, a dance they shared that they grew up with and had expertise in, to teach the class. A fascinating discussion occurred when White students shared in learning the Bachata partner steps that moving their hips during the partner dance felt sexually provocative for them. The Latina students took a pause, staring at each other in shock, and then countered, asking how the White students could feel comfortable rolling on the floor in their fan rolls, spreading their legs with their pelvises facing the audience but feel moving their hips in the Bachata choreography was provocative. It was a rich and respectful exchange between the students wherein the concept of cultural norms around flirtation, sexual innuendo, and propriety ensued. Both groups of students left with an understanding that the line of propriety in each of their cultures differed. Both groups committed to trying on movement from each other's cultural backgrounds.

This sort of exchange engenders discussions that illuminate distinctions between explicit and implicit beliefs and biases. This enriches the scope of conversations and perspectives in the area of observation and analysis. Cross-cultural dialogic exchange has the potential to diversify ideas and perspectives between students and instructors, adjudicators and dancers, etc. Not only does it expand the lexicon of movement and aesthetics for students, but it also increases empathy for varying perspectives and experiences in dance classrooms when careful attention is paid to the historical power dynamics that affect inequities between socially dominant and marginalized groups and identities in these interactions.

When I circle back to my ethnographic sensibilities to offer a frame for intercultural exchange, I see the potential and the power of dance educators as part-time ethnographers, taking a step away from imposing standards and toward curiosity and discovery of differing perspectives and cultures. From my personal experiences in making a concerted effort to remain open, nonjudgmental, and unimposing when it comes to my personal values and dispositions, I have come to a number of precepts that guide this state of being in the classroom and in cross-cultural settings in dance education. These are things I have developed and use in my own working ethnographic methodologies that also apply in the classroom when looking at dance works created by students that are a part of their cultural heritage and background:

1. *I (teacher/observer) am the outsider/guest.* I conduct myself as such. This means approaching my relationship to the work as one of a guest exercising the skill of empathic listening and curiosity instead of as a didactic expert.
2. *My opinion/perspective is not central.* When I am a cultural outsider to a form, no matter how long I have been present in the community, my perception, way of understanding, actions, and decision-making are informed by my previous socialization and cultural identity. While I can become more attuned to the sensibilities of the culture I am exposed to, I am always only one perspective that should be given secondary status to the voices of those cultural insiders.
3. *My perspective is not true.* Rather, my perspective is a proximal analysis or gaze that is separate from what truth is in the culture I am immersed in. What I understand to be true about my experience is only true of my experience, and those whose socialization and background align in a way that "rings true" for those with similar backgrounds. There are also people for whom my analysis may not resonate, as they may process a similar experience very differently based on their socialization and cultural background. In effect, my findings, points of discovery, and knowledge illuminate as much about who I am as they do about the cultural or dance experience I am engaging with.
4. *I frame thoughts as dialogue, not as final word.* The value of my discoveries and knowledge generation is in what I learn about the relationship between myself, the student, the student work I am engaging with, and my positionality in relation to the dance work, not in what I state as factual or accurate analysis of the dance work. My analysis is informed by the implicit biases generated from socialization mechanisms in my upbringing, education or training, and culture. For this reason, it is more generative, equitable, and culturally responsible to share from a place of self-reflection about my relationship to the dance work, both challenges and successes in that negotiation, than it is to attempt to describe, organize, or

articulate any structural truths or generalizations about the dance work.

These considerations for educators as part-time-ethnographers in examining the work of your students is crucial in creating a space for a more inclusive and equitable learning environment.

Another responsible alternative when working with dances outside of your area of expertise or cultural background is to hire experts of the dance form whose cultural background is that of the dance form the student is showing, if different from that of the instructor. With so many cultures and lived experiences, it is an unreasonable and impossible task to know in a full and intimate way the culturally relevant nuances and aesthetic orientations of each and every student that comes through our studios and classrooms. With an orientation toward dialogue and exchange between your knowledge systems and those of your students, students become agents of their own lived experience, called upon to articulate their position, biases, and the lived experiences that seeded these aesthetics and creative choices. This work takes a deep listening, openness, and empathy for the lives, perspectives, and creative preferences of each student.

One method of note for providing feedback in the dance field is Liz Lerman's Critical Response Process (CRP), a method that has been used in dance education for decades.[9] It is a structure that creates a clear and thoughtful environment and creatively useful structure where viewers can share their associations sparked from the work and ask questions of the artist. Artists can receive feedback and set boundaries about what they would like to know from the viewers. This process leaves open space for student observers to establish their own creative associations to dance works when giving feedback on what they saw. This structure for providing feedback on dance works deters any external influence by the facilitator or even of the choreographer that may influence or trigger implicit bias in an audience member's sharing of how they experience the dance work. The CRP's initial focus on audience members sharing what they notice, what ideas, sensations, or associations come up for them is a key component to disrupting the influence of personal biases that establish valuative statements about the dance work.

Another component of the CRP is the viewer asking *neutral* questions before the choreographer or performer specifies what they would like feedback about or whether they would like to hear personal opinions about whether viewers experienced a specific feeling or sentiment. For example, in a student choreographed dance work wherein the dancers face front the entire time, instead of the viewer asking, "Why didn't you do any turns or face different directions?" the viewer's neutral question may be something like "Can you tell me about your choices made relating to facing and spatial direction in this piece?" In this way, the curiosity shifts from an artist feeling the need to justify or explain something the viewer implies was lacking and shifts to the assumption that the artist is making intentional design choices to have dancers face the way the dancers face.

These two ways of engaging with students—initial impressions instead of evaluative statements and neutral questions—allow students to contribute perspectives that may go unrecognized if the structures for class engagement are too restrictive or prescriptive. CRP's tracking of neutral questions calls on the experiencer of the art to reflect before speaking. It requires viewers to practice distinguishing their personal values, which rely on assumptions about what they think the creative work *should be*, from genuine curiosity about the artists' intentional design choices and line of inquiry, research, and examination of their guiding content. Viewers of a dance work think before responding in order to separate out their personal biases from the artist's work. Then viewers examine what underlying assumptions might have motivated their initial sentiment. Finally, the viewer considers how to frame other possibilities relating to their experience of the work and pose dialogic questions that center on the artist's exploration, not the viewer's wants or expectations of the work. In this model of feedback, there is personal exchange between students and teachers, viewers of the work and artists on an individual discussion level, not a didactic critique of a student's perspective or individuality based on the stereotypes of student biases or pre-existing standards about dance that the observer may have.

This intentional consideration of personal implicit and explicit biases and how they function in a dance education setting should also be examined, not just within individual classrooms but at a programmatic level as well. For dance programs, it is important to explicitly track observational biases that may be prevalent in the program, as well as name the aesthetic or educational philosophies the program values. It is crucial to orient teachers to the norms, expectations, and standards of the program while also respecting the diversity of aesthetic and educational values that enrich the dominant perspectives in any singular program. The more explicit the explanation and description of the communal orientation, the clearer students, prospective students, potential instructional hires, and members of the greater community will be on what the program does well based on the programmatic orientation. Sharing these explicit programmatic biases helps move an institution away from the idea that a program meets all needs in some universal way. Making these biases more explicit also assists the program in better aligning curriculum and other programmatic choices to these values. More explicit sharing of values and perspectives also helps newcomers or those considering the program understand whether the program aligns with their own values or the values they aspire to.

One structural disruptor to implicit bias that can take place in the dance studio and also on a larger programmatic level is to no longer privilege those that come into the class with the most advanced technical proficiency. For students who have come in with technical prowess, they have had access to the financial supports and dance educators that could realize this goal, while other students may come with passion for dance, but without the same kind of access to the resources that would provide such training. It is important to disrupt a bias toward those students who have had access to extensive training. Privileging those with the resources to access such training reifies the systemic economic privileges and access to resources that are not equitably distributed across society. I, for example, now regularly assess engagement, ability to work with each other, ability to generate and communicate creative movement ideas efficiently and generously with each other, in addition to student growth in executing movement. This can be a policy or protocol in studio courses across a program should educators and administrators so decide. In studios and classrooms where executing what movement skills the instructor presents is a predominant model, this more inclusive assessment model also disrupts the assumption that the instructor holds the knowledge and the students replicate that knowledge.[10]

Qualitative Change in Assessment and Advising

Because so much of dance assessment is through visual observation, analysis, and interpersonal exchange, tracking and critically questioning whether perceptions align with reality or with our preconceived notions of a student are crucial solutions to disrupt bias. In addition to looking at the statistical data of grading, another check from the qualitative approach to how implicit biases may be showing up is to have an outside observer be an independent assessor. Inviting an expert in dance observation who has different aesthetic or pedagogical sensibilities or contextual experiences with students than you do engenders a rich potential to see a new perspective. A person with a differing perspective, who does not hold the same assumptions about what "good" student performance looks like, is an invaluable instigator to help unravel the "Yes, but why do you assert that?" and "What are you seeing or assessing that makes you think that?" questions that those of a similar background rarely raise. This second opinion of sorts is not meant to supplant your own final evaluation, but, rather,

6. Numbers, Qualities, and Bodies 151

to critically examine how you are seeing and what you are considering in evaluating student performance.

In addition to the recommended checks on implicit bias as it shows up in the dance studio, the following questions are a place to start addressing, naming, and establishing disruptors of implicit bias as a dance program or as an educational cohort of instructors relating to observation:

- What are some ways to track bias in observation in order to make it visible?
- How can teachers reduce the feeders of bias when observing students?
- What are ways to disrupt teacher biases once those biases have been brought into consciousness?
- Who is the support community that helps you see or track discovered biases?

In addition to clarifying the disruptions of observational biases, there is also aesthetic bias to contend with. Here are a number of questions for individual teachers and dance programs to consider in bringing into clarity the aesthetic biases in the classroom, studio, and social fabric of the educational setting:

- What are your goals for aesthetic clarity or consistency? How do you track those in a class?
- How do you balance the following in your classes?
    (1) industry or field standards
    (2) personal preferences
    (3) student clarity of their own creative concepts
- What are ways to illuminate aesthetic biases you may not realize you have?
- What ways can you "hardwire" into your class some comprehensive structures and methods of assessment that are not overrun by your personal aesthetic preferences?

Another area to disrupt biases extends beyond the studio into classrooms where history-, theory-, and writing-focused dance courses center canonical knowledge about the field of dance and dance education. Here are some questions to consider in devising, critically reviewing, and revising classroom courses in dance:

- How do you establish balance between the following in your classes:
    (1) standards in your field of study or in the culture of academics

(2) personal academic preferences
(3) the knowledge that students enter your class with?
- If the instructor is unfamiliar with content contributed to a class, what steps are taken to consider the rigor or accuracy of the content contributed?
- Is there space in your coursework or research process for students to examine how to incorporate knowledges not acknowledged or researched by academics or established artists?
- What protocols or practices can you implement in your classes to make your biases or the biases of your program, studio, or institution more explicit for your students?
- What are possible ways to clarify for yourself and for students when you are communicating a standard of the field, a personal preference, or an opportunity for students to articulate their preference?

Each area discussed above—observation, aesthetics, and systems of knowledge—can be examined at the individual level for each instructor or each course and at the program level. These components may also be exhibited beyond their most common environments where they manifest. Observational biases often show up in studio technique courses. Aesthetic biases often show up in creative process and composition courses. Knowledge biases often are prevalent in history and theory courses. This does not mean that each component does not cross-pollinate in other settings in a program. For example, there may be an observational bias in a theory course presentation or student group-led activity. I recommend being expansive rather than restrictive in examining where these implicit and explicit biases manifest in your educational setting.

Priming: Short-Term Change

In this section, I will focus on solutions that expose members of an educational community to priming tactics that disrupt implicit biases. Establishing priming measures that expose the person affected by implicit biases to counter-stereotypes to their bias is an example of a qualitative, contextual, community tactic that combats the negative effects of implicit bias. The intervention of putting up posters in a classroom or studio setting as mentioned earlier in the book is an example of priming. Priming entails exposing a person to unconscious, indirect suggestions that attune to the message the person enacting the primer intends. In the case of posters in the dance spaces, students are exposed to messages of what the teacher values, defines, appreciates, or deems inspirational about dance.

The research on priming and its effects on minimizing the influence of implicit biases suggests that even if a student is consciously unaware of the posters, the unconscious mind is affected by and attunes to the messages on the posters. This notion of priming can also work in the reverse in educators when they consider whether the messages on the walls of their studios and classrooms are contributing to an unintended implicit bias. If you notice that you as a teacher may be unintentionally priming your students in ways you do not intend, you may be able to effect change with the awareness of the significance of such priming methods.

Examples of other short-term ways to counter biases are to provide yourself as the instructor with short quizzes or regular, visual stimuli that run counter to biases you have. For example, if you have a negative bias against Black people, establish pictures in your home or office that depict Black people in a positive light and thus counter negative stereotypes. A more immersive and long-term solution would be to read books, watch films, incorporate media, or establish partnerships or routine social events that immerse you in positive experiences of those you have a negative bias against. These debias techniques to "prime" the perceiver are temporary when not applied long-term and must be reinforced. The computer screensaver example provided in Chapter 5 is an example of this technique. This solution of exposing a person to short, visual images in passing that counter the implicit bias provided by Banaji and Greenwald also resonates with Moore and Yamamoto's assertion that expanding movement experiences develops a fuller movement lexicon of possible meanings in analyzing movement.[11] These suggestions from Banaji and Greenwald's work illustrate that priming can be effective for both the implicit biases the educator may already have and the implicit biases students may have.

Syllabi are a potential site for priming students and for examining manifestations of your own implicit biases as instructor. Review syllabi and course planning with the goal of disrupting implicit biases and becoming more aware of explicit biases you know exist as the instructor and that the students exhibit in class. Syllabi often privilege the biases, perspectives, and values of the teacher. Examining syllabi through the lens of becoming cognizant of owning and naming implicit and explicit biases as the teacher and/or creator of the syllabi helps initiate a closer look at the teacher's positionality. This helps students understand the teacher's perspective as one perspective, not *the* monolithic or even most valued perspective of the dance field. It also helps students begin to discern where biases show up in the class and how to separate the personal opinions of the teacher from the salient concepts of the class material.

An examination of syllabi through the lens of biases can also help in the revision process of unpacking and disrupting places where biases present a skewed or narrow perspective for students. Another potential benefit of examining syllabi through the lens of where biases appear is to help disrupt any biases that may be counterproductive in the students. Are there stereotypes, assumptions, misconceptions, or misrepresentations students have that can be disrupted by amending the syllabus in a way that presents examples that counter those assumptions or expand student understanding of the dance field? Are there ways to alter the syllabus that upend the ideologies of U.S. oppression, exclusion, and misrepresentation, or even a teacher's personal fervor for ballroom dance, for example?

Amending syllabi can be a daunting task. In order to provide a manageable way to revise syllabi, I suggest exploring one of the following elements at a time so as not to overwhelm yourself as an educator and to make the changes most clear and effective in manageable portions. Examine one of the following at a time: (1) the conceptual or movement content covered in the class, (2) the artists or scholars represented in class examples and demonstrations, and (3) the pedagogical methods of interacting with students and structuring the course. Any of these entry points in considering biases (implicit or explicit) and how they show up in syllabi can effect change in assumptions, misrepresentations, or complicity in or reification of systemic biases or injustices in dance classes. These categories of syllabus revision can happen one at a time, for example one semester in content, the next semester in representation, etc. Another structure is to think of one change and its ripple effects. For example, think of adding one artist from a historically marginalized group in dance for the diversification of representation, and how that addition can engender change in the content of the course and pedagogy of the class around this one artist. Of course, there is also the radical approach of blowing up the entire structure for a full overhaul of a course in response to the culturally specific and programmatic needs that best serve all students.

Because implicit biases are undergirded by implicit memories, creating new lived experiences that run counter to existing implicit memories has the potential to supplant older implicit memories with newer ones created from newer lived experiences. The more opportunities to counter existing implicit biases, the more likely the negative effects of implicit biases can be deterred. Culturally relevant teaching is a crucial component of undoing implicit biases.[12] This teaching method calls on the educator to include representations, examples, and references from the cultures of their historically marginalized students in the classroom instruction. When educators are intentional in including culturally relevant examples and resources in their classrooms, they create new lived experiences that can supplant the implicit memories that students have received. It is a disrupter to the implicit biases that signal to historically marginalized students that they are not included in the narratives, histories, and stages of dance educational settings. This disruptor also offers a change in exposure to both stigmatized and dominant students and artists in the environment alike that marginalized members of society are present, valuable contributors, and full members of U.S. society and the field of dance.

Having content in the curriculum that does not represent historically marginalized groups of people both represented in the dance program and in society at large is damaging both to marginalized students and to students that are in groups at the dominant center of societal norms and standards. Bringing in content that is representative of marginalized groups of students in the class that are also historically marginalized in society, empowers these often-disenfranchised students to see themselves included in the field of dance with options to be successful. With no visual representations of dancers that are from the identity markers of historically minoritized students or the recognition of the contributions of those from historically marginalized backgrounds or identities, the message received is that the minoritized students are not part of the community and are outliers or out-group members that do not belong or are not fully appreciated or understood in the community.[13]

This intentional representation of marginalized groups in class also benefits the socially dominant community members in the dance program. It disrupts the assumptions that they are at the center. This tactic provides evidence and fodder for implicit memories in the unconscious brain-body of a different version of reality, where underrepresented and marginalized dance artists and scholars are evidenced to be talented, skilled, fully engaged members of the dance community. It provides an alternative narrative to the messages received that the field is only for dominant in-group members. It normalizes the belonging of marginalized dancers as members who, in fact, exist and have professional lives, contributing dynamic and rich work in the field. It is of note that many have not been exposed to the works of marginalized populations in dance.[14] Dominant culture implicit biases are effective in reifying the narrative that marginalized artists are of a separate category and are not central, iconic examples of the White heteronormative, thin, non-disabled-body dominant narrative that exists in dance.

Even if there are examples of dancers that are part of the pertinent marginalized population represented, there may be continued harm in how those dance examples are positioned in the curriculum or in programming. If dancers and dance scholars from marginalized backgrounds are only displayed either performing narrowly in culturally specific dance forms or settings, or displayed only as assimilating into predominantly White or other socially dominant structures or aesthetics, this can contribute to cultural cloning and should be avoided. It is important to do the work of researching historically marginalized groups of dance performers, choreographers, educators, and researchers to integrate them into current curricula to disrupt patterns of exclusion and implicit messaging. Admittedly this integration of diverse and inclusive resources may not happen overnight, but can be added in each iteration of the course or program until the representation of diverse groups is robust. Remember that this is an ongoing practice, not a finite goal with a singular point of success.

Other examples of methods that address long-term immersion practices that reduce unwanted biases against marginalized students include the "wise feedback" model described by Eberhardt.[15] This approach orients instructors toward the high expectations of students. It communicates to students that an instructor is giving feedback because the instructor knows the student is capable and talented enough to accomplish the fixes, even when society may have inundated both the student and the teacher with presumptions of the student's deficit or inferiority. In this approach, when feedback is given to students, teachers incorporate language that either explicitly states or implies the teacher has confidence that the student is capable of success. Of course, there is a thin line between sincerity and patronizing or communicating inauthentic sentiment. With a conscious awareness and persistent, tenacious reflective practice from the teacher that critically questions the language or behaviors tied to biases, this method can be a meaningful practice. This is distinctly different from the model of support that presumes and relays a deficit model to students that leaves students feeling as if the instructor has little or no expectation that they will be able to succeed on their own abilities, capacities, and intellect.

Eberhardt described her reflective awareness in a class she taught at San Quentin State Prison. When it came time for Eberhardt to return corrected papers the incarcerated men submitted in her class, she talked about struggling to find the balance between providing them with necessary feedback for their writing to improve while also not extinguishing their enthusiasm for writing. Eberhardt began to explain to the students when the class asked whether her Stanford students had a hard time receiving feedback: "When you have people who are used to getting positive feedback their whole lives and you tell them something different...."[16] She was then disrupted by noticing how the students were amused by this difficulty. Eberhardt continued to reflect on this moment: "I was trying to brace them for something—negative feedback—that had been a fixture in their lives. Criticism was a way of life for them. They couldn't understand why I felt compelled to shield them from harsh honesty"[17] She provided the example of a student's response to his paper covered in red ink corrections: "'I just can't believe it, [...] Somebody sat down and spent all this time on my paper, thinking of what would make it better and how I can improve. That's never happened to me before.'"[18] This immersion into the San Quentin State Prison classrooms and communities offered a different experience with a different community for Eberhardt that both called on her to maintain her high standards and helped her to understand the perspectives of a new, marginalized group of learners who were capable in ways that were unexpected for Eberhardt.

Community

Earlier in this chapter, I suggested finding colleagues that have differing perspectives or backgrounds in dance than you do as a resource for having critical and engaging discussions that may disrupt long-held assumptions and implicit attitudes. This is but one way to consider and engage with the larger proposed solution of developing community around disrupting the negative effects of implicit bias. Critical to the notion of developing a creative learning environment that disrupts the negative effects of bias is the ability to hold multiple perspectives in mind and to discover ways in which to hold each perspective in an equitably valued relationship from one perspective to another. This relationship is not one that can be tacked down, defined, or formulated without emerging from the spontaneous developments within the classroom and studio interactions and in discussion with other colleagues. No matter whether the community you gather together consists of you and students in your classes or you and other colleagues, the process of growth must include developing trust in the group; honesty with yourself and others; and openness to new perspectives, missteps, and discoveries about yourself and others. It is a practice in which the negative effects of implicit biases will inevitably occur. The work is to engage in communication that reveals harms caused, identifying manifestations of implicit memories and socialization, and to track bodily sensation to regulate feelings that occur in these exchanges. For educators, this means the role is to help in creating an environment of curiosity, discovery of connections and possibilities, as well as to support the class or cohort of fellow educators in the journey toward the common goal of honoring each member as part of the generative process. This is a whole improvisatory practice where new community, practices, and ideas emerge from a collective instead of in solitude.[19]

Educational philosopher and scholar Maxine Greene centers creating knowledge from the interstitial spaces that exist between dialogue and imagination.[20] There are a number of scholars who speak about this creation of knowledge through collective, shared engagement.[21] This is a different way to think about how knowledge is created than the singular scholar orientation. In this model, knowledge is not just thought of as only living in a written text or digital format, in one central, formally sanctioned, vetted, or approved space, but, rather, in the space between people exchanging ideas. This perspective considers how knowledge lives and is created in the exchanges between people. The perspectives, when shared within the context of imaginative possibilities and civic responsibility, can generate new ideas, ways of thinking, and creative systems that are born only from the space of the exchanges. Greene articulates,

> When we relate all this to the acknowledgment of the newcomers in our country, our cities, our classrooms, we come to realize (or ought to come to realize) that there cannot be a single standard of humanness or attainment or propriety when it comes to taking a perspective on the world. There can only be ongoing, collaborative decoding or many texts. There can only be a conversation drawing in voices kept inaudible over the generations, a dialogue involving more and more living persons. There can only be—there ought to be—a wider and deeper sharing of beliefs, an enhanced capacity to articulate them, to justify them, to persuade others as the heteroglossic conversation moves on, never reaching a final conclusion, always incomplete, but richer and more densely woven, even as it moves through time.[22]

Not only does this model of acknowledging and creating knowledge move past a single standard approach for learning, but it also calls for an ongoing dynamic for which the process is a practice, not a singular protocol to meet or funnel into one singular viewpoint. This model then "leaves individuals the liberty to transform the system."[23] In the classroom, this transformative liberty is built from an open space for a student's initial and authentic associations to come forth with the influences of educator's associations set on equally valuable footing as that of the students.

Students in an undergraduate dance education course I taught illuminated this open dialogic discovery for me. The class concept we were discussing was Elizabeth Gibbons' Guided Discovery and Convergent Discovery described in the Spectrum of Teaching Styles.[24] Gibbons writes that Guided Discovery happens when "the teacher uses a sequence of questioning designed to bring the learner along a path of discovery to a single correct answer."[25] Convergent Discovery happens when "the teacher presents a task whose intrinsic structure requires a single correct answer."[26] In this class discussion, I became concerned that students were struggling with what, for me, seemed to be a rather simple concept: the idea of guiding students to a single correct answer. Over a number of class sessions students continued to question me about this concept after I provided multiple explanations.

6. Numbers, Qualities, and Bodies   159

After some time, it became apparent that the issue that the students were struggling with stemmed from their immersion in a program that centered the inclinations of postmodern dance. The perspectives from faculty in their modern technique classes led to students struggling with the philosophical concept of what a single right answer actually means in the dancing body. After I celebrated and got over my exasperation at their deeper level of investigation of this concept (after all, I, too, have a postmodern dance bias), I explained to them that this questioning of the notion of a single correct answer was a testament to their exposure to a postmodern sensibility. I further explained that there are some learning contexts, such as the developmental needs of students in PK-12 learning environments, dance programs, or studios, that center on accuracy, established movement vocabulary and dance terminology, and detailed unison and conformity to specific phrase work in various movement techniques. Thus, the concept of a single correct answer may be accepted as a curricular standard that they would have to learn to adhere or adapt to as teachers, or at least learn to articulate their different perspective in a professional context. I had to explain to these students who oriented toward each individual's body exhibiting a different truth or individual embodiment of movement concepts that there were going to be educational settings where a tendu was a tendu or an undercurve was a very specific movement.

So, in this discussion, I explicitly named the bias in our dance program toward a more postmodern sensibility of movement and articulated that other segments of the dance community they will encounter may have differing ideas about this perspective and may value the idea of one single correct answer as a sensibility or even central tenet. In this class discussion, students engaged in a philosophical quandary that I had to catch up to. I left enough room in the conversation for students to share their answers to my questions without guiding them to a set of "right answers." Rather, I allowed them to share what the concepts in the reading meant to them and how they imagined these concepts taking place in the classroom.

In the end, allowing students to freely share their own personal experiences resulted in a vibrant exchange. In this exchange, students left discovering a little about their personal positionality in the field of dance that was developed in a dance program with postmodern biases. I left with a fuller understanding about how effective the curriculum of our dance program was at fostering a well-developed postmodern sensibility in our students, but with gaps in understanding what implications that may have outside of the university setting. What was most important for me as their instructor was helping them understand their perspective as one of many, not the singular correct perspective. In the same way that they did not presume there to be one physical right answer in dance classes, I also helped students understand this was also the case in the diverse approaches and sensibilities of various dance education settings.

Consider how rich the discussions, fuller understanding of various approaches, values, and perspectives in the field of dance education could be if dance educators met regularly and had similar discussions about defining features of dance and dance education. For this reason, creating long-term sustaining communities committed to disrupting the negative effects of implicit bias is another valuable solution. Bring together accountability partners that help deepen personal understanding of how your words do or do not align with your actions, that can call you on instances of equivocation that avoid taking action. It is important to have trusted partners and may even feel a bit uncomfortable hearing from trusted partners from different walks of life. If your quandary is in dance, I suggest not just asking people in the field of dance for support in this processing but to also include those who may not fully understand the field. It is in those moments that assumptions of the in-group of collegial dancers cannot nestle the questioner back into the safety and comfort of implicit biases.

One caveat to this is in examining issues that have aspects of sociocultural and historical marginalization within them. For example, if the goal is to examine a bias about race and you are a person of the dominant group, in this case a White person, I suggest not starting the discussion with a person of color. Seek out White people who have extensive knowledge and have invested in the process of unpacking their privileges as White people. This protects the marginalized group, in this case people of color, from being the recipient of further harm in your learning and growing process. It also prevents asking people of color to do additional work that is not their responsibility to do. In effect, marginalized people have enough to cope with in navigating their own marginalization in society. Do not ask them to add the work you are doing onto their pile of labor.

As the manifestation of bias, be it implicit or explicit, in dance curriculum may be challenging to pin down, creating a community of critical thinkers who provide feedback and support an educator navigating their biases is valuable. There are several ways that structured or unstructured community support can happen. One unstructured way is to form intentional communities to bounce ideas off of with people that you respect but who won't simply affirm your ideas without critical feedback. By intentional, I mean critical thinkers who can specifically address the area you would like to receive feedback on. These can be colleagues within your field, but it is also important to have members of this community of support be people who are not in the dance field or who may not even be educators. What becomes apparent in examining how biases work, is that part

6. Numbers, Qualities, and Bodies   161

of their ability to go unchecked is reified when we are surrounded by those who think similar to the way we think, that therefore affirm our way of thinking.

The exchange in Chapter 5 that I had with a colleague from the School of Education researching implicit bias illuminates the value of these exchanges with out-group members. Without this colleague's quandary on why implicit bias matters in areas that do not purport to be unbiased, I may have missed expounding on the implications of bias in the field of dance that in large part celebrates and makes manifest the voices, lived experiences, and thereby the biases of the creators and contributors to the work. At times, it is valuable to hear the thoughts, interpretations, and questions of outsiders to dance education in order to check any assumptions that are normative or commonplace amongst a community of dance educator colleagues.

The benefit of connecting to a critical questioning exchange with those outside of your in-group is exemplified by the graduate level teaching courses I developed. I was charged with combining two graduate level courses designed to prepare incoming graduate students for teaching undergraduate courses at the institution. One course was originally designed for dance graduate students, and the other was originally designed for theater and design graduate students. The theater course included students studying in the history and theory of theater and performance studies in the MA/PhD and MFA students studying costume design, scenic design, lighting design, and projections and media design. Instead of focusing on the nature of the specific content each student would teach, I centered the class around questions of pedagogy, curriculum-building, and disrupting negative effects of implicit bias in the classroom. Part of the activities for the course involved meeting in small groups with those in your same area of study. Other times students were asked to meet in small groups with classmates who were not in the same area of study. In this way, students were able to get feedback from those knowledgeable about their area and also understand how to better translate—concepts like weight shifts, and kinesphere, in the case of dancers or backlight and pinspot for lighting designers—to those who had no background in their area of study. Classmates unfamiliar with the content being covered in the lesson planned could articulate what was intelligible and what was ambiguous as a novice learner in the subject matter. Classmates from the same area of study were able to provide suggestions for structuring material, resourcing examples to illustrate concepts, and methods to deliver the content or better meet learning objectives. Having students from different academic areas of study come together to support, critique, and learn from each other's teaching approaches was a richer learning experience than keeping students separated by area of study.

Beyond the classroom, in other selection and evaluative processes in dance education, including dance experts from a different area or genre of dance is also beneficial in encouraging implicit bias disruption. There currently is little structure or recourse to check and identify ways in which the selection committee-gatekeepers are of a particular group-aligned bias. The more varied the aesthetic preferences and dance backgrounds of the selection committee, the more likely it is that assumptions of any one person on the selection committee can be identified and unpacked for any harmful, inequitable effects on applicants. In moments where one evaluator perceives an applicant or auditionee's performance very differently than other evaluators, these moments are fertile ground for challenging, plucking up, and calling out any unspoken biases. This is done by asking for more explanation of why the evaluators perceive things so differently. I posit that instead of seeking out like-minded individuals for these selection committees, that the group of evaluators be both of the current system and also include evaluators of historically marginalized groups and backgrounds of the applicants in the applicant pool. For example, if there is a lack of representation of disabled people in the school or program, or of dancers from different dance styles outside of contemporary, modern, and ballet in the applicant pool, it is important to include in the selection committee members of the underrepresented community. This inclusion of expertise from a different perspective assists in challenging assumptions of those from similar backgrounds and offers up new ways of seeing and evaluating dancers.

Deeper and Broader Range of Empathy

A significant element of a successful community is empathy in community members. In the field of dance education, what kind of dance educator training must be employed to engender Moore and Yamamoto's strong urge to understand the Other? In what way are our training programs equipped to require students and educators in training to be open to understanding movement styles, contexts, and moving bodies that are unfamiliar to them? How rigorously are the dynamics of empathic responsiveness, inclusionary practices, and conceptual understandings of sociopolitical power structures assessed in order to maintain the integrity of a dance studio's credentials, a dance program's accreditation, a movement analyst's certification, or a teacher's credential? Part of the answer to the above barrage of questions is integrating critical theory into programs that involve assessing and analyzing dance from dance educator certification

6. Numbers, Qualities, and Bodies 163

and professional development programs, to dance programs, to movement analysis training programs.

The ability to see the dynamics of power as they manifest between individuals in the field, in our institutions, as well as in the cultural contexts of our researched movement environments is key. The idea that cultural variation dictates perceptual acuity or sensitivity is also important to consider.[27] In other words, we are unable to see what does not already exist in the brain-body as a concept. The educator's cultural background affords them certain well-developed perceptual abilities in some areas while other areas remain less developed or completely imperceptible. For this reason, the idea of training with expert dancers, educators, or movement analysts is only beneficial if the trainee is training under a number of varied experts from differing systems or backgrounds of expertise. This diverse collective of experts would include those who have unique areas of strength in perceptual acuity and/or those who are both cultural insiders to the environment being observed coupled with those unfamiliar with the environment.

In addition to establishing personal connections with those being observed, I assert that instead of similar backgrounds, the educator should focus on developing empathy and open curiosity with those they plan to teach and work with. If educators take steps toward breaking down the boundaries of their personal preferences and identities as experts, work to make visible and then set aside their movement and cultural assumptions of others, and develop an empathy of seeing movers as both unique and equal, educators can access a broader range of perspectives and subject matter as well as a fuller understanding of movement content. The resulting expansion of movement and cultural content, possible new vocabulary, and frames of reference increase the movement lexicon available to educators. It also disabuses the dance educator of expertise in notions of observer neutrality or universal elements of movement.

When working in community, in addition to empathy, personal reflection is a large part of the unlearning process when it comes to implicit bias. Returning back to my example of becoming aware of an implicit gender bias I shared in Chapter 5, the reflection process was a prominent part of the process in unraveling what biases were operational for me. What part of my socialization was fueling this imbalance? How was I thinking about the choices I was making that made my decisions seem logical and sensible? The class was a Somatics for Athletes class that consisted of a majority of male-identifying students in the class who were all on sports teams in the school. There were only two female-identifying students who were not on sports teams in the school in the class, and no gender non-conforming students. My assumptions about the male students in the room and about somatics was that socially, the male students may feel uncomfortable examining internal felt senses in their bodies and reflecting upon their own relationships to their moving bodies. My assumption was that the female students would not have such a struggle in attending to such things, as females had been socialized to do more of this internal processing than the male students.

To adjust for this assumption, I was making more efforts to engage the male students in the class, assuming the females would be more comfortable sharing and could jump in without prompting. Of course, the other dynamic in the room is having such sense-oriented reflective conversations with high school-aged students in a mixed-gender class. The female students did not engage regularly in this majority-male movement class. I also own the real possibility that what underlain my logic was pure internalized oppression as a woman who has been socialized to make sure males in my environment are comfortable, while the females are on their own or assumed to be capable of finding a way to be comfortable.

While this reflection was done mostly on my own, reflection does not have to be a lone endeavor. For a more structured approach to examining negative manifestations of bias in dance education, I offer the Critical Friends Protocol[28] as one example of a structured model for providing teacher-to-teacher support in the reflective process and getting feedback and ideas from other educators. This protocol is a structured way for teachers to share a specific dilemma or question they would like to hear responses about and receive feedback from a small group of fellow educators. This protocol uses order of activities and specific time limits to move in a productive way through a session that allows for each educator in attendance to receive feedback. The structure ensures equity of time dedicated to each member of the group, creative thinking and problem-solving within the group, and group collegiality of hearing the experiences, ideas, and challenges of other educators. Here's an abbreviated summary of the structure of this protocol: one group member steps into the role of presenter of their issue. For two to three minutes for each of the following, (1) the presenter shares their issue or question, (2) group members ask probing questions, (3) group members share affirmative feedback, and (4) group members share constructive feedback. Then for five minutes, the entire cohort has a discussion of potential solutions to the issue. Finally, for two to three minutes the group creates a challenge or action-oriented step addressing the issue for the presenter to take on. This process then repeats for the next cohort member to proceed through their 15- to 20-minute round of this process.[29] I participated in this protocol process during my time teaching in a high school as part of the professional development support in the school. My experience was positive in that it felt supportive, substantive, and gave me insights and new ideas about how other educators from other subject areas were addressing similar issues in their classes. For those in the cohort with me, it was a common occurrence for them to note their surprise at both the unique situations of dance classrooms and what we as educators had in common in the way of goals for best practices. This format also offered clear examples and evidence of the plurality of potential solutions to be garnered when educators come together.

Effective Other Models

Remember that singular options or examples in the limitless possibilities and social contexts of classrooms and dance studios are only minimally advantageous. There is no one right answer to solve the negative effects of implicit bias. Here I offer a few other resources to consider in creating more room for a multiplicity of voices, to remember and acknowledge power dynamics operating in community, and to disrupt the assumption that an instructor must be the sole source of knowledge in a classroom or studio. In Wernick, Woodford, and Kulick's case study[30] of an LGBTQQ[31] theater program, it becomes apparent that there is value in creating an intentional community wherein students become agents that promote inclusion, hold adults accountable, and normalize LGBTQQ lived experiences in schools. When examining the incessant messages of the societal power dynamics, it becomes necessary to create equally persistent counter measures that not only disrupt the misrepresentations that bolster inequity and exclusion, but that also foster methods of speaking up and making intentional change in the culture of the classroom, the hallways, the virtual spaces, and all other spaces. The researchers of the theater structure discuss how the combination of Performance Action Research, collecting data through surveys, and student-devised theater performances interspersed with the data helped adults understand the exclusionary sentiments, alienation, and inequity LGBTQQ students experience. This model combined the quantitative data collection with the students' qualitative creative process and shared personal narratives to effectively voice the marginalization students faced in their educational settings.

Another useful source from the theater community is the Theater of the Oppressed work of Augusto Boal,[32] a devised theater method that reflects the values and pedagogical approaches of Paulo Freire in his work on critical pedagogy. The practices and activities offered in this theatrical method calls on participants to examine the dynamics of power between actors, characters, and audience members. It not only addresses the structures of theatrical development, but also the potential perceptions of the audience members. One example from this approach is a tableau exercise. Students are asked to silently create a group still image that depicts power dynamics between the people in the tableau. Then another group of students suggests small changes to the tableau that would change the power dynamics of the relationships originally displayed by the first group. As students conduct a round of these tableaus, they examine how they interpret the power dynamics in the original tableau, and what may have changed about that dynamic when the tableaus were changed. In this exercise, it is not uncommon for students to interpret the power dynamics differently, while also learning to appreciate the creative choices of their classmates.

Embodied Solutions

In addition to quantitative and qualitative solutions to disrupting the negative effects of implicit bias, there is the third category of embodied solutions. This category of solutions is a starting place for how to think about possible practices that upend the negative effects of implicit bias that require attention to the body. This involves tracking internal felt sensations. It also involves developing an awareness of the effects of biases on surrounding environments, communities, and people and creating new habits, behaviors, and practices to upend choices based on those negative effects of bias.

Internal embodied reflection includes tracking sensations that well up in uncomfortable situations. These situations are potential sites and exchanges where biases are triggered and begin to inform interactions in counterproductive ways. Internal embodied reflection in these moments of discomfort involve assessing where practices do not align with personal intentions, self-perception, or programmatic goals or missions. These are the fleeting ephemeral moments dancers understand are as real as they are transitory. They are the behaviors and small, subtle ticks that signal approval, disdain, acceptance, or elitist division. These are the holding of tension in the body replicated, transferred, reflected, and echoed from the moments of tension taking place in the environment. This area of addressing the negative effects of implicit bias involves self-responsibility, ability to articulate and name the behaviors witnessed, and an ongoing and collective practice of deepening the attention to the embodied responses and interactions with others and the environment.

Brenda Farnell contributes to this discussion of the importance of bodily sensation in the observation process.[33] She speaks of the role of the sensate body in relation to objectivity in the context of dance ethnography.

Farnell reminds the reader that the myth of Cartesian duality, splitting the thinking mind from the feeling body, may delude participant-observers into believing either that their felt sense while moving, or the objective reasoning of their observation are sufficient in understanding the movement of another culture. She asserts, instead, that what the participant-observer experiences is an integration of sensation and understanding that is structured based on the metaphysical—how a person understands reality—and language structures of the participant-observer.

In dance studios and classrooms, this orientation can only be shifted after exchanges with the student population, which help educators understand the ways that students are orienting their intent and the meaning of the movement educators observe. In short, dialogue and embodied, felt sensation is crucial both in interrupting the perceptions of the educator as singular or central and in integrating a new way of seeing and understanding movement into the experience of the movement, i.e., into a new aesthetic sense Robin James articulates in Chapter 2.

For this reason, participating as a mover in the movement students share in class can be a valuable and relational method to physically empathize and understand the lived experience or embodied orientation of the student. It also models for students what openness to learning new movement looks like as an educator dedicated to life-long learning. A bit of caution, however: the balance in complexities is delicate. Participation should not recenter attention on the instructor, but should support full engagement of students through modeling behavior they should engage in. It is possible as an instructor, to take up too much space and attention from the engagement and work students are doing. This may take some time and effort to discern.

Another example of an embodied solution is encapsulated in the Activity Boxes throughout the book. In these activities, I ask the reader to stop and reflect on personal experiences, felt sensations in the body, or the courageous naming of the aspects living in the brain-body that do not align with the forward-facing external representation of who you are in the world. Much of this work integrated throughout the book comes from my personal experiences and practices in somatic movement practice and facilitation coupled with the work of somatic abolitionist practices.[34]

Tracking and attuning to the body in moments of discomfort, like those that occur with cognitive dissonance or when a bias is triggered, is one process Resmaa Menakem articulates in his work.[35] The practice is summarized as follows. First, settle the body through practices such as taking deep breaths or softening in your heart space. Next, notice the sensations happening in the body from physical or emotional feelings to any other sensations such as vibration or tension. Then, instead of attempting to get away from the discomfort, notice it as it is until you notice when the feeling changes to become a different type of sensation or feeling. After feeling this change, begin to engage in any response that is sourced from the better aspects of yourself. Finally, after the occurrence, if there is still some felt sense or energy of discomfort that lingers in the body, find a constructive and safe way to discharge that tension or energy. This can be done through physical movement activities like dance, yoga, walks, a sport, or even physical labor such as shoveling or chopping wood.

As with qualitative solutions, embodied solutions of this sort are important to also experience and engage within a community, not just alone. Moving not only alone but also with others is imperative in growth as it relates to dismantling the negative effects of bias. Engaging with others and developing these practices in a community that challenges perspectives you hold are important in expanding the scope of personal perspectives and in holding space for the values and beliefs of others. This is an ongoing practice, one that is about remaining attuned to and aware of what is happening in the brain-body as biases spark difficult or disruptive exchanges or experiences. After attuning to the occurrence in the moment, take a moment to reflect alone. Ponder what about this situation, this dialogue, this performance, or this student activity is inciting discomfort? Which assumption, value, or belief is it offending or calling into question? What relationship does that bias or association have to your sense of self or what you find important or central to the challenging situation? What harm are you imagining will come from this differing perspective or unexpected occurrence?

After managing and attuning to bodily sensations in the moment of the occurrence and reflecting as an individual, tapping into community to offer differing viewpoints is the point at which the importance of community comes into play. This can be people who understand and are knowledgeable of the circumstances, novices or outsiders who are unfamiliar with the context of the occurrence, or some combination of those. I do suggest if you are a person from a socially or historically dominant group, however, that when addressing difficult questions of bias as it relates to historically marginalized people, including considerations of race (BIPOC), citizenship status (non-citizens), disability (disabled bodies), body shape (thicker bodies), etc., first connect with group members of your own dominant assignation that are well-versed in the oppressive dynamics potentially in play.

People from historically marginalized or socially stigmatized identities often already have an inequitable, additional amount of labor. In their roles of support professionally, as well as in their daily lives, they do additional work managing the systemic power structures before even being

6. Numbers, Qualities, and Bodies

asked to have a potentially difficult conversation with dominant group members. Also, if you are from a historically dominant identity, there may be a power dynamic in the exchange that makes the marginalized person less comfortable or likely to be open and honest with you for fear of this honesty being misinterpreted as an attack that jeopardizes their status in the community. Asking them to do additional labor to assist you is not the most attentive way to initially consider these additional factors in play in community.

In considering how pervasive systemic oppression is in the socialization mechanisms of daily life, it is important to reflect upon how oppression affects community dynamics and, by extension, bodily behaviors when there is no intervention to disrupt the mainstream White, heteronormative, patriarchal, thin, and non-disabled-body orientation of societal norms and, by extension, the field of dance education. When there is no attention to how messages that support misinformation, disregard, microaggressions, or exclusion are taking place in a community, a passive community reinforces whatever cultural norms and systems of hierarchy and power inequities are operating in the normative socialization messages of U.S. society. In order to disrupt these sentiments and how they contribute to implicit biases, an intentional community must be built to counter, invalidate, and call into question normative assumptions about marginalized members of a community.

As with the dynamics of any community, the daily consideration of how a community is forming itself and reifying or disrupting pervasive social patterns of dominance over others, is complex and contextual. It is also an embodied endeavor, one that happens to stigmatized bodies and through bodily behaviors that affect the community. Each community must consider what is needed for their specific community and consider how it is displayed through bodily behaviors and how it is experienced by others in the community. This attunement to the cultural dynamics of any dance community often goes unnoticed as we carry our bodies around both exhibiting behaviors and experiencing messages from the community in each interaction within that community. In order to develop a practice of affording space for every body, every person, every history of lived experience in the room, this fleeting subtlety of power made manifest in bodily behaviors must be addressed explicitly.

One way to explicitly address what sharing space for every student and/ or educator body looks like in a community comes from a practice I have in my own classroom and workshops. I support a classroom commitment to embodied and behavioral authenticity by asking students to create a set of community norms at the beginning of the semester. Depending on the size of the class, my familiarity with students, or their familiarity with this activity, I sometimes start with a set of norms that I have collected from a number of different sources.[36] Other times, I have students create these norms completely on their own and then use the community norms list I devised as a check to ensure students have everything they need on the list.

What is important is that these standards are created in collaboration with the students. If there is something on the community norms list that I devise that students don't feel is particularly pertinent or relevant, then it stays off the list. The list is also a "living" list, meaning that should things need to be amended, based on student requests or issues, the list can be adjusted as the term progresses. These norms sit at the intersections of qualitative interpersonal dialogue in creating the norms and an embodied practice in honoring the norms through behavior in community with others.

Activity Box #14:
Ongoing Integration and Reflective Practice

For at least one week (if possible, a longer period of time like a month or an academic term), keep a list of personal biases, aversions, and priorities that come up for you in your daily life. As you begin to collect this list, can you rank the items on the list? What organizational system or qualification did you use to rank the instances? Under what circumstances might the items change positions on the list of priority? How might these items in your list connect to your past experiences, memories, or cultural backgrounds? Are there ways that these items are aspirational, that are about progressing toward a different belief than you carry from your past? As you collect these biases, track any ways that decisions, behaviors, language, and thoughts either confirm or conflict with the listed biases. Where are you in alignment with your stated biases? At what moments are you in misalignment, wherein your decisions, behaviors, language or thoughts are not consistent with the stated biases? Are there moments that align with one bias but conflict with another bias?

When engaging in this activity, take time to track sensation in the body and move, if possible, in a way that reflects your new entries and connections each time you write in this journal activity. If available, over the duration of your ongoing journal collection, create a community of others interested in participating in this activity. Arrange set check-in sessions where you each share what changed or came up for you in your ongoing list and reflections. When possible, share movements that resonate or reflect your discoveries within this group sharing.

7

Reintegration
A Fuller Picture

For a fuller picture of how these concepts look in a dance studio or classroom, I offer a more integrated narrative description of solutions to the negative effects of implicit bias based on examples from my dance education settings. These examples provide a fuller context of how I implemented techniques that disrupt implicit bias in my classrooms and what they could look like in your classrooms. The first section outlines ways to explicitly state your cultural norms, values, and positionality as a teacher in an effort to name your personal biases and lived experiences, placing them as precursors to what is to come in the class. The next section furthers the process of getting to know members of the classroom through identity explorations in a Laban Movement Analysis course. An embodied exercise further extends this process of getting to know one another through embodied empathy and attunement in a composition class. The following section offers an example of helping students organize their thoughts about theoretical concepts explored in theory courses to inspire more dialogue in class and writing beyond class sessions. In the section about how to integrate conversations about bias into history and theory courses, I provide both cursory questions I use in my class discussions as well as a more comprehensive approach taken from Dr. Karen Clemente's history class. The final and most comprehensive example is taken from a middle school dance curriculum I developed to address social inequity and implicit biases both in student research outside of class and embodied practices inside the classroom.

Positionality and Explicit Classroom Norms

In my own classes, after the obligatory syllabus review, I then shift to what the students would like to see happen to create an environment that supports their learning. For this I introduce the notion of explicit community norms that were discussed in Chapter 6. Again, depending on student familiarity with this concept, I either ask students to create a list of classroom norms from their own ideas or I present them with a starting list of proposed examples.[1] I explain to them that this starting list is just a proposed list of ideas that they can either accept or reject. Next, I talk through each item on the list to further describe what its implementation might look like in the classroom. After hearing from students what needs to be amended about the list, I then explain to them that this list can change if needed as we go through the course. If I am in a PK-12 setting, I usually have the community norms listed on a large sheet of paper or poster board for students to reference throughout the course. For higher education settings, I simply share it as a document to access alongside the syllabus.

Then, I shift to sharing a bit about my own personal biases so that students have a sense of my background and biases. I often state my personal value systems around student learning. In this discussion I also acknowledge my personal bias toward challenging the existing assumptions and power structures flowing through the U.S. and, by extension, the academic and art worlds. I share my values for critical thinking and consideration of positionality. I explain how bias shows up in wonderful ways that help us understand each other, but also in unintended ways that assume or expect others to have the same opinion. I regularly playfully explain to students that it is *extra credit* if they can share with me the points of class content that they disagree with or that aren't true for them. I encourage students to dialogue and share their perspectives, even if those perspectives are ones that I do not agree with.

My focus is on the practice of students articulating those ideas, not on whether I believe them to be right or wrong. I celebrate students who can articulate their point and relate or contrast their point of view to others in the class including me. Then, when pertinent, I point students to resources or areas of study that help them support, substantiate, or deepen their own perspective. For example, I had a student who wanted to create a dance work about disabled dancers but was not planning on including actual disabled dancers. Because she was a non-disabled dancer, I kept mentioning and suggesting the importance of including the voices and experiences of disabled dancers if this was what she wanted to explore. She continued to forgo my suggestion, citing the difficulty of finding disabled dancers. I then found a resource I mentioned in a class feedback session that crystalized the issue in the statement "Never about us without us."[2] The student was able to read the resource and find more creative ways to include the voices of disabled dancers in her research and her dance via various quotations and sound and video recordings with an acknowledgment that substantive growth would have been deeper if disabled dancers were collaborators in her process.

I sit in a space of curiosity when responding in the discussions for classes, as Greene's work inspires educators to do. In these dialogic exchanges, I ask questions for clarity, propose examples of what the student describes to determine whether the example aligns or not, and describe possible sticking points to the veracity of the position to determine whether the student's statement applies in differing circumstances. This practice positions students to be more sensitized to the grip of fragility, to better track when they feel harm or offense and how to manage it constructively during class discussion should a person disagree with them or their perspective.

Critical thinking also allows for students to consider more possibilities than the singular truths of one author, artist, or resource. It implores students to think that even though this is one example of a concept, it is not a standard by any means as there are a multitude of ways a concept can exist, operate, manifest, etc. I also name if it is a standard for a subset of the dance community to help give a fuller perspective of where the field of dance is in relation to the conversation.

Identity Exploration and Laban Movement Analysis Activities

Another useful area of exploration in dance spaces is identity exercises. These identity exercises help students connect their personal lived experiences, memories, and identities to their personal biases. For example, when teaching Laban-Bartenieff Movement Analysis, I begin with an identity exercise to help students understand how their personal identities and socialization relate to how they perceive and, therefore, how they analyze the world. There are a number of these exercises pulled from a number of equity and inclusion activities and exercises I have done in past professional development work.

Flower Power[3] is one well-established activity in which each petal of a flower represents an aspect of a person's identity. For each petal of the flower, a student enters their identity in that category and then shares their flower creation with the class. In more recent renditions of this activity some of the formatted categories include race, socioeconomic status, spirituality/religion, age, gender identity, literacy level, immigration status, education, etc. I think it is important to incorporate in dance communities how students identify their body image and physical ability, as these two categories are rather significant in the way of stereotypes and access relating to success in the field of dance.

Another exercise for identity exploration in the classroom is a writing assignment that poses the question "I am from…."[4] This activity is a written activity where students have a poetic prompt structure to speak of the foods, geographic location, languages, and people they are from. After completing the written portion, students then share their activities in small groups or with the class as a whole.

An additional activity called "Who Are You?" is a more embodied activity with no writing required. This activity works well in studio courses where students are less likely to have a writing utensil and paper handy. Students are arranged in pairs. For a full two minutes, one student asks their partner, "Who are you?" Each time the other student answers, it must be a different response that shares additional information about who they are. Students then change roles to repeat the exercise.

After completing one or, if there is time, a few of the identity exploration activities in the Laban-Bartenieff Movement Analysis course, I ask students to either look over their written exploration of identity or think through their answers shared in the verbal identity exploration exercise. In thinking through their own identity and their relationship with dance and understanding of movement, what might their system of movement analysis include? What elements of movement would their system focus on? Are there elements that are a significant part of their identity or their relationship to movement that they would incorporate that they feel aren't considered in their formal education about dance? Are there elements of dance or movement that are talked about in their studies of dance and movement that would not be a major component of their own system?

This is usually a reflective assignment I introduce during class. Then, in order to give them time to think deeply about what the system might look like, I ask students to continue working on it outside of class and to share in the next class session. At the end of the semester, I return to them their submission of what their system would look like and ask them to consider if anything of their system might change based on their work in the course. This activity is meant to consider other options that do not center one system over the possibilities of other systems. I also may incorporate resources that speak of the Laban-Bartenieff Movement Analysis system in comparison to other movement analysis systems such as Ann Hutchinson Guest's comparative scholarship.[5] These are ways I contextualize one analysis system as one perspective, developed within the cultural contexts of its creators with the open possibility of students having their own voice or perspective based on their own culture.

Empathy, Attuning, and Implicit Bias: A Composition Activity

I was asked to come in to teach in an introductory composition class with special attention to my research on implicit bias. In this class, I decided to focus the 50-minute session with a class of approximately 20 students on the relationship between empathy and implicit bias as evidenced in the social science research. This session considered the claims that implicit bias can affect our capacity to show empathy for another person. After detailing what implicit bias is and how a disaffinity with a person can reduce the level of empathy for that person, I asked students to consider two aspects of this information in the context of developing movement. One element I asked students to consider was what their own personal biases were that affect their creative decisions and choreographic dance work. The second element I asked them to consider is as a person learning movement material, how might the ability to empathize and identify with the mover affect the ability to embody nuance and detail of that movement.

After framing the class session with these two questions, I asked students to use a writing utensil and paper to draw a circle on the paper over and over without lifting their writing utensil, noticing how that circle and their bodies change as they repeat this movement gesture. After doing this drawing activity for a minute, the students showed their paper to the class and shared any reflections they had on the sensations that happened in their body as they drew on the paper. Next, I explained that this is how I would like them to embody the next activity.

Then I asked students to think about a bias they have and to develop one movement that reflects that bias in some way. I told students that they could choose a bias they felt was insignificant or unimportant, such as their favorite color, one that felt important to their identity or opinions about dance, or one they felt was an unpleasant or problematic bias. After developing that one movement, I asked students to repeat that same movement but with an open exploration of how the movement then morphed, traveled, and changed as they repeated it in a similar way as the drawing activity. The movement could change minimally or as drastically as transferring to a different body part.

After the students had some time exploring the movement, I asked them to pair up with another student. Once paired, one student would begin to move this repetition score while the other students would "attune" to movement they observed. As students moved, I clarified that they should think about attuning as energetically different from mimicking. Mimicking is shape-based, focused on ensuring things look alike. I asked students to think about not just the visual shape of the movement but the energy, theme, and feeling of the movement. What are other details, nuances, and aspects of the movement that repeat? What elements shift with every repetition? These are the questions that guided this partnering exercise. Partners then switched roles to explore for three minutes for each partner's turn.

After these two explorations, students were asked, without talking to each other, to develop a way they would combine the two movements into one short movement study to show. As they began to work on this silent coordination, I asked students to be mindful of the choices they were making of how to coordinate. What were their choices in how to communicate combining the two movements? Because the class was large, these explorations were very short to leave time for student sharing, but both the individual and partner explorations could be extended based on the time allotted in class.

If time allowed, I would have had students engage in feedback through the Lerman Critical Response Feedback process I often use when helping students develop the skill of providing substantive feedback to the artist.[6] Even in using this set structure, after having some time engaging with the pre-established version of the feedback protocol, I challenge students to think about what is working, what is most beneficial or pertinent, or what is needed for particular moments or situations that they may want to amend or change about the feedback protocol. This way, students get to engage critically with the structure not as the final word or indisputable rule of thumb, but, rather, as a guide for them to then engage in their own personal decisions around how to incorporate what they find valuable.

In addition to the feedback process for the movement shown in class, I also held a discussion with students where I asked them to reflect on their decisions, creative choices, and felt embodied sensations as they moved through the class activities. In this discussion I asked questions about what tendencies or biases either in the body or in the choices made did they notice making. In working with their partner, did they notice a tendency to lead initiating a structure or did they pull back until their partner started first? I also asked students to examine how they understood what it meant to *attune* in their bodies. In embodying the concept, how much was about synchronizing in timing, in shape, in quality, etc.? If there were any reflections on empathy and the ability to *see* each other and the details of the movement, those would also be valuable, though they tend to be a bit more of a challenge in the vulnerability of that level of reflection. This might also serve as a written reflection after the class session ends.

Praxis of Dance Theory: Getting to Writing

In theory courses in the classroom, one structural bias often built into theory and writing-centered dance classes involves privileging students who can interpret, integrate and communicate abstract and theoretical concepts quickly. For those who struggle with contributing to class discussions or in writing, I often suggest a more physical and creative solution to ponder the theoretical concepts. One of the most meaningful and powerful models for processing theoretical content from my own days in graduate school was the task of creating a metaphor of what I understood of the theory. A predominant way that Dr. Penny Hanstein, contemporary of Maxine Greene and chair of my MFA dance program, asked students to share their analysis of course readings or concepts was on large sheets of paper. We students were asked to draw the relationships between concepts and how they related in some larger metaphor. Instead of asking us to process in linear, physically disembodied ways, she asked us, as burgeoning dance scholars, to think about what experiences we know about life that could be the metaphor of how the main ideas, concepts, or theories related to each other. This enabled those who cognitively come alive through drawing, story-telling, or physically moving and manipulating ideas to contribute to the class discussions in deeply creative, nuanced, and personally meaningful ways.

Take, for example, the concepts of theory and embodiment. These two concepts could coil around each other like snakes either in struggle or in mating behaviors as a metaphor. Maybe for some, theory sits atop embodiment like whipped cream that slowly melts into embodiment, or maybe theory lives inside of the concept of embodiment with theory as the viscera and embodiment as the bones or skin. There are limitless, creative, and conceptually rich ways for students to then think about, discuss, and extend course concepts in robust ways that don't simply replicate another person's perspective. The level of depth and capacity to think the metaphor through in detailed and extensive ways supplemented class assessment beyond the number of times a student may have contributed to the more improvisational component of the discussion. As individual students share, both classmates and the instructor may ask questions of clarity that invite the creator of the metaphor to more fully realize the detail and fit of the metaphor to how they understand the concepts.

Addressing Bias in Dance History, Theory, and Writing Courses

In writing-centered classes, after sharing my positionality and values in a class, I incorporate specific ways students can practice this tracking of bias in class reading and writing assignments. For example, after reviewing a class reading and emphasizing the salient points that I want to make sure students attend to, I ask the students questions such as the following.

- What are the biases of the author?
- What type of dance, movement or aesthetic philosophy, population, or area of the field of dance does the author center their discussion on?
- What circumstances, dance forms, populations, etc., are left out of or not considered in the reading?
- What does the author, artist, or reviewer spotlight and what is left out of that focus?
- What is useful and not so useful about this resource for you personally?
- Who or what does the content apply to and who or what does it not apply to?
- What are some assumptions the author, artist, resource makes that are not explicitly stated?

Dancer and scholar Dr. Karen Clemente presented a poignant and more comprehensive way to address bias in a transformative presentation titled "Bylines and Bias Part II" at the 2016 National Dance Education Organization Conference.[7] In this presentation, Dr. Clemente sourced and demonstrated the arc of how to incorporate dance critic reviews of African American dance performances in a 20th- and 21st-century U.S. modern dance history course. Through this process, her primary source demonstrations of various reviews illuminated the patterns of racial bigotry and bias that were apparent over time right up to contemporary sources. This presentation stuck with me for years after, as it made real and apparent the structures and operational power of racism in the field of dance. This presentation also validated my own personal experiences of how some dancers, scholars, and critics steeped in tropes of Whiteness speak about, critique, and assess Black dancers and their creative work. Using primary resource materials of critic reviews and, when available, performance footage of the dances reviewed, this course put Black dance and Black voices at the center of the conversation while critically examining the systemic dominance of Whiteness that devalued the work, its significance, and the value of and contributions to Black dance in 20th- and 21st-century U.S. modern dance. While Dr. Clemente was presenting on this material as early as 2013, this conversation still endures in more public venues.[8] This presentation is a testament to the challenge of movement, action, and creative innovation relating to unending racial bias in a field that so often sings the praises of its capacity for movement, action, and creative innovation. While moving through established canonical ways of thinking about U.S. modern dance history, this course also evidences the residual, pervasive, and malleable yet perpetual hold that socially constructed biases like race have in our perceptions and our lives. I contacted Dr. Clemente for more information about this curriculum, and she graciously provided further information about her class.

In Dr. Clemente's Modern Dance History undergraduate course, students pull back socially normative veils to see the patterns of application and immersion of racial biases in the messaging and employ methodical processes to research that serve to disrupt these biases. In her course, Clemente offers assignments where students find critic's reviews of early modern dance pioneers and asks them, among other questions, to track and describe the biases in the critics' writing. She asks in one assignment, "Were there biases or assumptions made about the Postmodern era of dance? If so, describe."[9]

This is a question that I ask of students now no matter the publication. I ask this question so that students can begin to locate the positionality of the author and name the biases present in the author's work. I do this not just to develop critical thinking skills for students, but also to help them determine which positions they affine with. Who are the scholars, artists, educators that align with their own perspectives and why?

Dr. Clemente then continues in this assignment by asking students to view the work that the critic is reviewing whenever possible. This way, the students can view, from their own perspective, primary source material of a moment in contemporary history and how they experience that work today in comparison to the critic's perspective. Having students analyze and articulate their experience of dance works on their own terms while also comparing and contrasting their experiences to that of critics is another strategy that helps students locate their perspective in the sea of dance artists, scholars, and educators. Dr. Clemente continues this methodical approach to unpacking bias with questions like "Was an appropriate context (important background information) provided for the work?"[10] Analyzing the critic's claims in this way allows the student to examine how the sociocultural and historical context of the dance work affects the critic's perception of the performance. Clemente then deepens the critical reflection process with questions such as "What stereotypical language was used?"; "What assumptions were made?"; and "What information was missing?" Dr. Clemente includes examples of the type of information omitted, invisible, or disregarded such as context, details about the specific type of dance, and whether experiences of African American perspectives or aesthetic traditions were considered in the critique.[11]

Through this process, Dr. Clemente is directing students to the practice of disrupting the processes that socialization may have made invisible. Specifically, she illuminates the epistemic biases of Whiteness to separate Black creative work, both artistic and scholarly, from the cultural context of the work's creator and often from the predominantly White canon of dance works. This decontexting shifts the comparison of the work away from the existing dance form and its internal rules and logic, and instead compares it to the norms established by Whiteness, and thus disregards or invisibilizes the aesthetics and perspectives of people that developed and consume the work. Not only does Dr. Clemente help make this new operational racism visible through first person resource materials on dance critiques, but she also helps students develop practices, research methods, and analytical techniques that guide students in the critical and discerning process of naming racial biases and racists patterns of perception in the analysis of dance.

Middle School Creative Process Dance Class[12]

The final and most comprehensive example of my attempts to disrupt the particular negative effects of implicit biases in my dance classrooms comes from my experience teaching a semester-long middle school social justice unit. The context in which I originally developed this curriculum was in a small, predominantly White, private school dance program. The cultural context of the school was one where the school explicitly stated a commitment to social justice for students. Dance was an elective students could choose from among other elective class options.

I then modified the curriculum in other school settings based on classroom dynamics and ages, including elementary school (fourth–fifth grade), high school, and college levels. The program settings were often at schools that did not have dance as a mandatory class for all students resulting in a wide range of talents and abilities. Some students were curious about what it would be like to take a dance class, while others were studying up to 16 hours per week in competition dance studios. While the student population of the schools where I taught was predominantly White, I did have a significant number of students of color consistently hovering anywhere from 10 percent to 40 percent, primarily from Black, Asian, and Latinx racial identities.

In the initial iteration of this curriculum, there was only one dance class option for middle school students, so students interested in dance had to be together in one class for the grade-level meeting once a week, and then they also met with all of the middle school dancers, grades six to eight, once a week. No matter the grade level, students met twice a week, once with their grade level only and once in a combined class of all sixth–eighth graders enrolled in dance.

The structure of the dance course when I first began teaching at the school, however, was explained by fellow colleagues and students in the course as one with a hierarchical, social dominance orientation (SDO). In this orientation, the "trained" students with access to technical dance training were privileged, and the students with no dance training were marginalized. To disrupt this culture of privileging those with technical dance training, I flipped the role of leader and follower, having the students guide the focus and subject matter of the choreographic content, while I served as facilitator and space-holder to support student goals.

In the way of content, instead of introducing movement concepts I found standard in my canon of concepts for class, I introduced concepts that allowed for student voice and collaboration in choreographing as a group via the language and concepts of the Laban-Bartenieff Movement Analysis system, as well as research content in the work of social justice. With regard to representation in the class, I brought in guest artists who aligned with the movement genres that the students were investigating and using to create their work. Of those guest artists, I was mindful of bringing in underrepresented artists who disrupted student experiences of White women being the predominant dance teachers.

I changed the dance class model from a dance technique-centered course into a choreography-centered course. Instead of learning the basics of ballet, modern dance, and hip hop, students spent the semester choreographing dances based on their personal interests in those dance forms and their interests and experiences of social injustice. This de-centered the expertise of those skillful technicians in the class who took dance up to 16 hours per week and opened opportunities for success and leadership to students with no previous dance background. Instead of front-loading predetermined movement for students to be assessed on, I as the instructor-facilitator provided class warm-up and movement phrases that helped in student performance of the movement they were creating. This centered the developmental scaffolding of movement and the evocative exploration of choreographic ideas that supported the final phrase work students developed once students began to develop movement and choreographic ideas. If students developed movement in a dance genre in which I had no experience or expertise, I brought in guest artists who could support student work in this style, providing both technical support for the movement and feedback on their execution of their choreographic work.

Students were not only agents of their own creative process; they were the generators of the movement content from which the class was assessed. This structure allowed the opportunity for those with little dance background to substantially contribute to the class through deep critical thinking, as well as an ability to communicate in an effective and supportive manner with fellow students. This also disrupted the assumption that dancers are only well-versed at physicality rather than a wide range of skill sets.

Allowing open discussion and organization of the decision-making process also brought the element of challenge and social negotiation into the classroom, where dynamics of oppression, power, and privilege occur. As instructor-facilitator, it was my responsibility to gently guide; question; and, when necessary, help students identify stereotypes, biases, and microaggressions, or any other unintended or unnoticed disregard for students who are marginalized in some way. This is where I, as an educator, was responsible for making visible the manifestations of implicit bias I could see happening in the interpersonal, social dynamics of the class. Naming implicit bias, supporting students feeling excluded, and helping students learn to see those moments for themselves and have language for them was another mechanism for disrupting the negative effects of implicit biases. The way in which I examined or called attention to these moments were through reflection questions and gentle openings in the conversation that created space for the non-dominant voices to speak and share their feelings, perspectives, or lived experiences. These conversations were not oriented around good or bad behavior, appropriate or inappropriate contributions established by me, but rather on facilitating discussions that addressed empathy and learning to hold to the class goals of making a stellar dance while also tracking how students were affecting each other in positive and negative ways in the process. This class was another place where I invited other educators or administrators into the room to offer me their perspective as it relates to any negative effects stemming from my own implicit biases that I may have been enacting in the classroom dynamic.

Sorting through solutions of how to structure the curriculum, I decided to focus on the creative process as a site of learning for all students no matter what level of experience with dance they may have. It had been my experience that most dance studios taught various dance techniques

7. Reintegration

but generally did not provide classes on how to choreograph dances. I therefore organized the class around content that I hoped would level the field of expertise between students with extensive studio experience, students who loved dance and knew dance in their own social contexts, and students with no experience of dance classes or experiences of dancing in their communities at all. The notion of having auditions does not align with my value that everyone should be welcome and has something to contribute to the creative activity prospects of dance, nor was it helpful in sorting out student capabilities in the creative process. Deciding to forgo auditions in this class also served to reduce the anxieties around student's technical levels of expertise and reduced the competitive ethos of the class.

The semester-long structure I provided was for the class to develop a final dance work that addressed some area of social injustice to be performed at the end of the semester for classmates and parents. Goals and assessments were oriented around level of engagement and understanding of the creative process; ability to complete incremental tasks that built into the final dance; ability to work collaboratively, creatively solving problems with classmates; and ability to reflect on this process. Through this structure, I choose to shift more of the decision-making process and location of responsibility for holding knowledge in the classroom from me to the students. I was the facilitator guiding students through the process with a healthy round of instructional details that framed structures, plans, and guiding questions. Instead of orienting the classroom to a curriculum where I choose the choreographic content, I helped the students to determine the subject matter and the aesthetic they would like to embrace in their collaborative dance performance event.

In my first year, I shared with the students this shift toward articulating their ideas to each other in description and planning of movement composition activities and in directing others in how best to execute their creative ideas. I did this in an explicit way, explaining what was important from my set of values and what I was looking for and evaluating students in the class on, while also acknowledging that the frame is simply a different approach for which I have a bias different from their previous instructor. With a number of the students coming from competitive studio dance backgrounds, the shift toward choreography and personal voice for students who collectively had minimal experience in articulating their own ideas through movement evened the hierarchy of student skills.

In the construct I created, making decisions in this classroom community was different from having students vote or having the teacher making the final decision. Instead, the decision-making process was based on what I call the *consensus* model of finding the connecting aspects of a theme or concept that relate to some part of each idea contributed. This consensus model of collaboration is about a mutual agreement amongst group members that each person's ideas and interests are included at a level that is acceptable for each group member. This process, instead of a majority-rules model, requires students to restructure the ways that ideas, concepts, and goals are interrelated and speak to each other. In the context of the democratic process in the U.S., it is less like voting, where the majority rules, and more akin to how congressional bills are made to contain just enough of each perspective at an amount that is agreeable to all legislative authors.

In order to help students orient to this way of thinking, I introduced the consensus model concept in the class with a game I call "Combs and Kangaroos." This game, provided as an Activity Box in Chapter 1, was first introduced to me through Maxine Greene's protégé, Dr. Penny Hanstein. In this class structure it serves as a priming activity to disrupt socially pre-established categories already present in the minds of students such as shape, size, color, etc., and also serves as a reflective practice to help students become more intentional about creating new ways to categorize or couple ideas. At every moment that a group decision needed to be made, the class first played Combs and Kangaroos. Then students brainstormed individual possibilities, grouped the possibilities using the approach framed in Combs and Kangaroos and began to distill what elements could live together, be combined or relate, be applied for each decision in a way that the group has consensus about the combination.

It also, with some facilitation from me when needed, helped students practice not staying silent if they felt their ideas or perspectives were not quite present enough and helped avoid one student having final and full representation in the ideas and decisions. Students could now propose solutions that integrated their ideas more fully into the collective idea without getting rid of or diminishing the ideas of others. For example, when I teach this course, students often come up with the connecting concept of exclusion as the theme that connects each student's concept of inequity. With exclusion as the umbrella theme that connects each student's ideas, they could work deeply on their personal connection to this concept—i.e., body image bias, inequity in climate change effects, socioeconomic class disparities, and gender discrimination—while still holding space to find creative connections and overlaps with the ideas of others in the class.

The consensus community model employed in the course furthers the work of André Lepecki and Randy Martin with regard to dance being a mirror reflection of the real world and its sociopolitical topography.[13] When students are working with each other, they are working within the socialization paradigms that organize the structures of cultural biases, even if they have no conscious ability to articulate those biases. Having students engage in a semester-long creative process that requires them to share their ideas, make decisions, and integrate each other's voices into one singular dance work provides multiple opportunities for students to track power dynamics. For example, students might consider whose voice is most prominent in the process or in the group and why. Through questions and reflection activities, I assist students in tracking their own role and relationship to the group and help them identify the implicit biases and memories or experiences that underlie those relationships.

The first portion of the class was focused on introducing students to the Big 8 of identifiers that are socially constructed in the U.S.: race, socio-economic status, sexual orientation, ethnicity, religion/spirituality, ability, gender identity, and nationality.[14] This starting point had a couple of goals. First was to introduce the idea that creative processes and more traditional research would be partners in this process. Another goal was to provide initial information and content for students to understand the larger structures in place that feed inequity in the U.S. An additional goal was to provide clearly defined options of where to begin their own research that were both focused and clearly defined enough to understand, but still broad enough for students to relate to in unique and personal ways. For example, students could apply gender inequity to the lack of representation of women in high-ranking professional positions or to the discrimination of transgender people in a world that privileges cisgender people.

This information and list of options to begin their research served as a structured way to begin the discussion about social injustice in the U.S., with options for students to research and potential sites of interest for them to determine what they were personally interested in making a dance about. The general topic also held space for the consideration of equity and inclusion in the dance-making process itself. Not only were students tasked with making a dance about social justice, but they were also tasked with embodying social justice practices and maintaining their community norms in their creative and collaborative work making the dance.

Not just for this course, but for most of my teaching I share with the students that the type of learner I attempt to privilege is the learner who is proactive in their own learning, making their own active decisions in the learning process even at the risk of being wrong or passing the threshold of assumed standards about how the learning should manifest. I identify examples for students of the more passive banking model where students expect to receive all information from the instructor and then replicate or parrot it back to the instructor during evaluative events.[15] When those happen—for example, introducing the students to Laban concepts to help them have language to use in communicating with each other about dance—I explain that this is only one way the class will employ learning. There will be other moments in the class that the students will be asked to find new knowledge that I, the instructor, do not have and share it forward in the class. In these times, I ask students to pursue their own passions, to live into their own personal biases in order to follow them to further understanding about content presented in class and develop their own perspectives. This was the pedagogy to which this class was oriented.

Because I centered the way in which students were holding space and contributing to the community norms and connective tissue of the class as a whole, my general pedagogical bias was for students to have a shared responsibility for creating a space of learning. To communicate the expectation of this level of engagement, I either shared the idea or included the class article, "From Safe Spaces to Brave Spaces,"[16] for students to read to emphasize the need for risk-taking over maintaining comfort to promote learning and deeper understanding of each other in the class. I encouraged them to check in with and support each other, to negotiate and navigate what their boundaries with each other were, and to communicate challenging or vulnerable personal truths in service of learning about the lived experiences of each other. So, the value system of the class is oriented towards connectivity, creative adaptation, risk-taking, accountability to each other, and commitment to personal and class goals.

The measure of assessment in this course included the thoroughness of action and engagement in decision-making on the students' part. It was important to reserve judgment on the density or complexity of the knowledge gathered by students. I found moments to acknowledge to students that I had epistemic biases for what constitutes knowledge that align with the cultural norms of dominant culture. This modeled for students openness and vulnerability to the learning process and the need to question the rigor of resources.

For example, a student may have researched and collected knowledge about a dance form that either did not look like knowledge to me or seemed insufficient or underdeveloped, because the systemic support for archiving knowledge for the content may not have aligned with the structures I am accustomed to. A student's research on a dance form that does not privilege written histories but rather embodied histories where one would have to travel to griot-type figures to attain the knowledge may feel sparse to me. In this situation, I would guide students through a reflective process of where they looked for the knowledge (i.e., what efforts did they make to collect information); how far down the proverbial research rabbit hole they went once they found information (i.e., how extensively did they follow the referenced resources that would allow them to find additional resources); and if there were dead ends, why?

I emphasized to the students that I asked them to search for their own knowledge because they will be the new generation of knowledge creators. Then I shared that I wanted them to begin the practice as soon as possible to improve and advance the field. I actively and intentionally reserved judgments on the nature of the content and focused my assessment on the process of searching for the knowledge and presenting what was found in a thoughtful and organized way. This decentered my own personal biases about what acceptable or substantial knowledge content was and engendered students to follow their own path around the search for deeper understanding and learning while also asking critical reflection questions about the knowledge sources.

There was a moment during class where a student with prior dance training who was particularly locked into perfectionist visions of her work was teaching her phrase to a group of classmates who did not have the technical skill to execute a movement. When she had her classmates share the phrase in the class, she expressed her frustration at them not being able to fulfill the movement she created. Another student who also had significant dance experience prior to the class responded to her classmate's frustration, encouraging her to rethink the choreography and how to express the same sentiment through movement that would *look good* on the dancers while still revealing her main idea. This felt like a moment of success for me. The moment was a formative assessment moment where it was clear that students not only understood my perspective and expectation for creative development and collegial support in the class, but also were thinking about the ways that it could serve as a solution that met the needs of both choreographer and performers simultaneously.

Throughout the decision-making process, I, as facilitator, through reflective questioning, tracked and called to awareness when implicit biases may have been affecting who is heard in the room and whose ideas are being dismissed. Regarding their growth in physical and aesthetic development as dancers, I facilitated the physical and aesthetic articulation of student movement ideas through warm-up and phrase work material that strengthened and reinforced the work the students were developing. As students created phrases, I observed both the movement they created and the qualitative information about how they envisioned it being performed. From that information generated by the students, I created developmental movement phrases and large movement phrase work that supported student physicality of their movement ideas. For example, if I saw that a student was struggling with getting her classmates to travel in their phrase, I would integrate pelvic shift elements into the warm-up material, sometimes in a general way and other times in the specific movement of the phrase created by the student.

It was invigorating to hear students exclaim in class, *That's from my phrase!* Again, this was a formative assessment moment where I could track how and when students were able to identify movement ideas, concepts, and developmental patterns carried over from their work into the warm-up and phrase work I created. I would occasionally ask, "Now, why do you think I asked the class to do that last phrase I created?" in order to determine whether students were doing the internal work of connecting anatomical and technical movement concepts to their creative phrase work. Students remained engaged in deepening their creative work and in the conceptual discovery of developmental movement patterns that supported the work they were creating in the class. I would occasionally catch a student using part of a warm-up I created to prepare students to continue the work in a phrase that related to the warm-up phrase.

This curriculum incorporated Sensoy and DiAngelo's research in creating a framework for introducing and reinforcing student knowledge of social justice issues that are at the root of the semester curriculum.[17] This curriculum introduced a progressive classroom approach to learning the elements of dance that moves away from methods of teaching dance technique from a place of authority and toward student-centered learning.[18] Lastly, this experience introduced the idea of the body itself as a site of political protest in the classroom wherein students were encouraged to take agency over what their bodies expressed and were challenged to most effectively articulate those ideas physically and in group discussions.[19]

The feedback process in this course included a combination of the processes experienced from my participation in The Field organization's Fieldwork[20] process and Liz Lerman's Critical Response Feedback protocol.[21] These two approaches include room for viewers to respond based on their own personal connections and background rather than a specific formalized modality or predetermined aspects to respond about. This leaves room for connections viewers made that may not have come up had the discussion been initiated by pre-established structures or categories to look for or respond to in the movement.

For the student observers of the movement, this protocol entailed a clear process of providing feedback. The creator of the work got to define specifically what they sought feedback about. This was a wonderful way for students to exercise and reflect upon their interests, focus, and goals for the feedback rather than the instructor organizing that focal point. Another salient element of the Critical Response Process is the notion of responders or viewers of the dance work delineating valuative statements and questions from analytical statements and questions. This exercise helps students begin to organize their thoughts in a way that does not privilege their personal attitudes or biases about the work. Rather, this method

7. Reintegration

actively subverts the viewer's personal values about the work and recenters the conversation on the artist's intended area of focus for the feedback session. This feedback process also encourages respondents or viewers to share ideas and associations they have in viewing the work rather than sharing personal values about what the viewer enjoyed or valued about the work. Instead of evaluative statements, the Critical Response Process emphasizes the relationship between the viewer's personal associations sparked by the dance work and how those relate to the goals the artists have for the feedback session at the time of the showing.

Part of the cumulative assessment involved a reflection process via short video interview clips of each student answering a series of reflection questions I devised about their experience of the creative process. Questions encouraged students to reflect on challenges and successes in their creative process, interpersonal dynamics in group collaboration, and personal habits and practices. Students were also asked about which aspects of their abilities in the creative process they discovered were an asset and which were a difficulty. I then took those short clips and edited them into a pre-show video I shared with the audience about the creative process and what students organized and learned about themselves, each other, and the creative process. This is part of the process of learning the skills of deep listening and holding space for the ideas, personalities, and values of others in order to work together to create.

This change in approaches turned out to be more disruptive for the adults than for the students. Students were loquacious in sharing their ideas and perspectives in the class while supporting each other's opinions and feelings. They were so deeply engaged in the choreographic process, there were times where students reported to me their plans and needs for the day with the level of detail of any educator mapping out the needs and schedule for their own lesson planning. There were passionate debates where students each spoke how they felt about the subject and common sessions where students would stay after class sometimes just to hang out. Other times they shared something they were struggling with, were proud of, or had questions about in the class. This happened with both extroverted dominant personalities as well as shy social out-group members or newcomers to dance.

While fellow arts colleagues and my immediate supervisors who observed my classes were in full support of the intentional and inclusive approaches to the dance class, some parents and more distant adult members to this process were a bit more perplexed by the idea of centering a dance class around the process rather than around pristine product creation. The dances that students created were works they were proud of, that they shared with and invited their friends to, and waxed poetic about their newfound areas of knowledge about being an artist who not only performs but also choreographs. There were poignant responses to the student performances by audience members, complete with tears from educators, administrators, and parents at seeing a raw expression of the personal interests and passions of the student performers.

But of course, the response was not a uniformly positive response. There was also a palpable resistance to the aesthetically radical choice to privilege student clarity in design, coordination, and clear expressivity over technical prowess and superhuman feats of flexibility, uniformity, and technical execution of familiar dance vocabulary. I heard protests via students and messages sent through administrators from parents who had invested in extensive dance training for their children that they had strong objections to the approach and change in values. This is a testament to the power of the intimate connection between aesthetics and social hierarchies. For those that perceive art as an expression of a level of socioeconomic status and elite tastes, the concept of art being accessible for and to everyone can feel like an anathema to their defining features of art. Again, everyone has and is entitled to their biases. Dance educators and learning environments at large must examine the relationships of the biases we carry to systems and cultures of oppression, hierarchical dominance, exclusion, and inequity.

In Celebration of Bias: Embracing Egalitarian Thinking

As a final reflection on bias, I would like to back out a bit further from the deconstruction and dissection of ideas to better understand them and specific examples from studios and classrooms. I return to a reintegration and celebration of who we are as dancers and as educators in this moment. It is important to remember that art by definition is very intimately connected to bias. The creative process is one of indulging in one's own personal preferences, habits, decisions, dispositions, identities, and personal life journeys in order to speak to some personal expression about humanity and the human experience. It is relaying that personal vision to other collaborators in the production of the work who help the artist bring expression or personal sensibilities and attitudes to fruition. As with the creator and performers of the dance, so, too, with the audience. What an audience member connects with, attunes to, or even is disgusted or humored by is also an expression of their personal biases, some explicit, some implicit.

This book is not about stifling this intimate and creative process, but rather about reveling in deep, critical abandon and connection with others around this creative work. It is about standing in the truth of one's perspectives, passions, and processes without imposing those onto or demanding the same sensibilities of others. It is about sharing a perspective rather than establishing it as *the* perspective, about delving into one's creative self to learn more about who you are as an artist and educator and the ways you find your discoveries are aligned with or in opposition to how you know yourself to be. What happens when your personal voice integrates with and encounters the experiences of other collaborators on the project or in educational communities? How does that relationship affect the sensibilities of your own personal vision and biases in dance education? What is the attuning process when some aspect of your perspective does not inspire the sentiments you intend? These are the benefits of the reflective process in examining personal biases. There is a momentous capacity for discovering a fuller sense of self in looking at instead of suppressing biases and a limitless potential for finding common connections with and deeper understanding of others. To name biases discovered in the creative process or within educational systems as singular, unique perspectives rather than demanding they be a standard truth for the masses is the benefit of bias in the creative work of dancers and educational work of dance educators.

This also applies to students or contemporaries of any artist or dance educators and dance scholars as well. Take time to celebrate and more deeply discover your love for a teacher, scholar, or dancer's work without hardening the boundaries of their individual creative path or intellectual and pedagogical perspectives as the only or greatest path for the masses. As humans, we have the capacity to change over our lifetime, to grow in or out of love with dances and artists as we move through life. Now that you have become aware of how implicit biases affect our work in dance education, there is a responsibility to address any harm caused and celebrate clarity of our own perspectives in service of inclusion and equity in dance education. Take charge of regulating your somatic experience when triggers of cognitive dissonance occur or when challenged on harms caused. Allow breathing room for those shifts so that you remain malleable and perceptive to change and new opportunities for growth, discovery, and clarity of your perspective in relation to others. This is why I deliberately articulate the goal in this book to be disrupting *the negative effects of bias* instead of ridding a person of any bias at all. I assert that biases in and of themselves are not the problem, but rather a part of the human experience hardwired into our evolutionary path. The danger lies in the intersections of sociopolitical and socioeconomic power structures that influence human assumptions about what is a bias and what is a truth.

So as a dancer and educator in the world, continue to explore, expand, challenge, personalize, and create new paths from any ideas shared in this book. Test activities or practices offered here. Personalize and critique what is shared. Only through this relational process of sharing and engaging new perspectives can this work on how implicit bias manifests grow. Finally, celebrate your biases as your own personal perspective, as part of a dynamic growth process, and part of your life's journey. Find the balance of honoring the perspectives of students, colleagues, artists, and other stakeholders in dance education with a humility and acuity for equity, empathy, and inclusion that prepares for the inevitable missteps but expands dialogue, understanding, and human connection.

Appendix A
Social Justice Curriculum Design Outline

Planting Seeds: Social Justice in the Choreographic Process

Phase	Creative Process	Social Justice Application
Seed: Select Focus	Brainstorm and come to a resolution on topic	Decide what you choose to interrupt in terms of oppression
Plant: Clarify/Research Focus	Deepen understanding of your relationship to topic	Learn more on what you are drawn/called to set right or better for others
Germinate: Connect to lived experience and ideas	Transform ideas/research into personal intention	Seek your place within various communities and organizations that address the issue(s)
Sprout: Take action/Create	Develop phrases of movement/Compose/Expand through action	Do your work! Create a community and ongoing practice.
Prune/Water: Feedback	Give and receive feedback	Listen to the voices of others in the work.
Grow: Deepen & Expand work	Adjust actions and plans based on feedback	Adjust accordingly
Landscape: Frame your personal message/voice	Choose and arrange your perspective on the work for an audience	Become clearer on your place in the work as to serve your best purposes.
Harvest: Rehearse (relive) & Reflect	Continue to live your experiences more deeply and clearly with more clarity and reflection	Continue the work with reflection and re-clarifying your place best served in the work
Replant: Share with others	Perform your frame of reference for audiences	Share your experience/voice/passion with others beyond/outside of the work.

Appendix B
Community Norms Sample

Community Norms[1]
- Be fully present (stay engaged).[2]
- Participate in the discussion to the fullest extent of your ability.
- Speak from the "I" perspective (speak your truth).[3]
- Be self-responsible and challenging.
- Listen, listen, listen, and process.
- Lean into discomfort.
- Take risks, expect missteps as a necessary catalyst for learning.
- Accept conflict and resolution as a necessary catalyst for learning.
- Be comfortable with silence.
- Suspend judgment of self and others.
- Be crisp, say what's core.
- Treat others' candidness as a gift and respect confidentiality.
- What is said stays. What is learned leaves.

Chapter Notes

Preface

1. This is a term to refer to the physical skin-color signal of White people that does not necessarily align with the light-skinned person's way of identification. Because race is a construction imposed on people even before individuals self-identify, self-identification unfortunately matters less in the construction of race. However, in this instance I also had several conversations with my fellow travelers where they identified themselves as White as well.

2. Airhihenbuwa, Collins O. "From 1619 to COVID-19: A Double Pandemic." *Health Promotion Practice* 21, no. 6 (2020): 857–858.

Introduction

1. Relles, Stefani R. "A Call for Qualitative Methods in Action: Enlisting Positionality as an Equity Tool." *Intervention in School and Clinic* 51, no. 5 (2016): 312–317.

2. As a somatic practitioner, I believe the mind is an integrated awareness of the brain and body. For this reason, I use the term "brain-body" when referring to the mind to distinguish my own sensibilities from the mind-body dichotomy that operates in Western Cartesian sensibilities. When a study or area of research is specifically speaking about the hard wiring of the physical brain tissue, I will use the term "brain."

3. Kolber, Jerry, and Bill Margol. *Brain Games*. Directed by Michael Simon (October 9, 2011; Los Angeles: National Geographic Channel, 2011).

4. The term "glitch" has been discussed and problematized in a number of ways as connoting innocence, harmlessness, or lack of responsibility of the offender when there are such harmful ramifications of the negative effects of implicit biases. There are well-established cases made for there to be responsibility taken for the negative effects of implicit bias for offenders that address issues with the notion of using the term "glitch" seen in Negowetti and Mason; Holroyd, Jules, Robin Scaife, and Tom Stafford. "Responsibility for Implicit Bias." *Philosophy Compass* 12, no. 3 (2017): e12410; Levinson, Justin D. "Forgotten Racial Equality: Implicit Bias, Decisionmaking, and Misremembering." *Duke LJ* 57 (2007): 345; Mason, Elinor. "Respecting Each Other and Taking Responsibility for Our Biases." *Social Dimensions of Moral Responsibility* (2018): 163–184; Negowetti, Nicole. "Implicit Bias and the Legal Profession's 'Diversity Crisis': A Call for Self-Reflection." *Nevada Law Journal* 15 (2015): 431–460.

5. I would like to acknowledge the assumption implicit in the research that "the brain" refers to some normative standard of brain function, and does not speak to or account for neurodivergent variations of how implicit bias may function differently in neurodivergent brains or events. Malcolm Gladwell does provide a brief discussion in the conclusion of *Blink: The Power of Thinking Without Thinking* about autism and implicit bias; Gladwell, Malcolm. *Blink: The Power of Thinking Without Thinking*. Little, Brown, 2005.

6. Moore, Carol-Lynne, and Kaoru

Yamamoto. *Beyond Words: Movement Observation and Analysis*. Routledge, 2012.
  7. Moore, *Beyond Words: Movement Observation and Analysis*, 49.
  8. Sloss, Daniel, dir. *Daniel Sloss: X*. 2019; Sydney, AU: HBO Max, 2020, https://www.hbo.com/specials/daniel-sloss-x.
  9. For further reading and consideration of the role of memory, particularly in racial trauma, see Resmaa Menakem's work on generational trauma and decontextualized memories in the body.
  10. Payne, B. Keith, and Bertram Gawronski. "A History of Implicit Social Cognition: Where Is It Coming From? Where Is It Now? Where Is It Going?"
  11. Banaji, Mahzarin R., and Anthony G. Greenwald. *Blindspot: Hidden Biases of Good People*; Beeghly, Erin, and Alex Madva, eds. *An Introduction to Implicit Bias: Knowledge, Justice, and the Social Mind*. Routledge, 2020; Eberhardt, Jennifer L. *Biased: Uncovering the Hidden Prejudice That Shapes What We See, Think, and Do*. Penguin, 2020.
  12. Fricker, Miranda. *Epistemic Injustice: Power and the Ethics of Knowing*. Oxford University Press, 2007.
  13. Levinson, Justin D. "Forgotten Racial Equality: Implicit Bias, Decision-making, and Misremembering." *Duke LJ* 57 (2007): 345.
  14. Harris, Cheryl I. "Whiteness as Property." *Harvard Law Review* 106 (1993): 1707–1791.
  15. https://www.census.gov/quickfacts/fact/table/U.S./PST045219. Accessed January 4, 2020.
  16. This data was sourced from the Bureau of Labor Statistics for the year 2019, the Census Bureau for 2019 and from DataUSA.io for the year 2018.
  17. It is also important to remember when collecting data to be mindful of how the data is combined. In some of these sources of data, there were clear class and racial divides within one category. For example, here, the judges were combined with "magistrates and other judicial workers." Based on the Federal Judicial System data provided on the Americanprogress.org website, however, when the judges are separated from this more general category, the representation of Black judges specifically is a lower percentage than the percentage of Black people in the general U.S. population (https://www.americanprogress.org/issues/courts/reports/2019/10/03/475359/building-inclusive-federal-judiciary/) ; Adelstein and Bannon,"State Supreme Court Diversity," n.p.
  18. Where Is the Diversity in Publishing? The 2019 Diversity Baseline Survey Results. https://blog.leeandlow.com/2020/01/28/2019diversitybaselinesurvey/#:~:text=Gender%3A%20The%20survey%20reveals%20that,self%2Dreporting%20as%20cis%20women.
  19. Again, due to how problematic categorization can be in aggregating data, I have separated out the professions that required a medical doctoral degree from those that range in training from certificates to bachelor's degrees to master's degrees. I then sourced the specific numbers for each medical specialization from www.datausa.io.
  20. Sourced from https://datausa.io/profile/soc/police-officers#demographics.
  21. Sourced from https://datausa.io/profile/soc/dancers-choreographers#demographics.
  22. Higher Education Arts Data Services. Dance annual summary: 2018–2019. Reston, VA: National Association of Schools of Dance, 2009.
  23. For a snapshot of this conversation a decade prior to this publication, see Julie Kerr-Berry, Ed.D., "Progress and Complacency: A 'Postracial' Dance in Higher Education?" *Journal of Dance Education* 10:1 (2010), 3–5, DOI: 10.1080/15290824.2010.10387151 (accessed May 28, 2021).
  24. Davis, Crystal U., and Jesse Phillips-Fein. "Tendus and Tenancy: Black Dancers and the White Landscape of Dance Education." In *The Palgrave Handbook of Race and the Arts in Education*, pp. 571–584. Palgrave Macmillan, 2018.
  25. Fentroy, Chyrstyn Mariah. "My Experience as a Black Ballerina in a World of Implicit Bias." *Pointe Magazine*, June 5, 2020. https://www.pointemagazine.com/chyrstyn-fentroy-2646155391.html (accessed December 4, 2020).
  26. Howard, Theresa Ruth. "Op-Ed: Why We Need to Confront Bias in Dance Criticism." *Dance Magazine*, August 3, 2017. https://www.dancemagazine.com/op-ed-we-need-to-confront-racial-and-cultural-

biases-in-dance-criticism-2468342343.html (accessed December 4, 2020).

27. Spears, Courtney Celeste. "How Dance Students Can Confront Racism and Implicit Bias in the Studio." *Dance Spirit*, June 10, 2020. https://www.dancespirit.com/students-confront-racism-2646167153.html (accessed December 4, 2020).

28. Williams, Riis. "Ballet Bias." *Real Change*, July 15, 2020. https://www.realchangenews.org/2020/07/15/ballet-bias (accessed December 4, 2020).

29. McCarthy-Brown, Nyama. "Owners of Dance: How Dance Is Controlled and Whitewashed in the Teaching of Dance Forms." In *The Palgrave Handbook of Race and the Arts in Education*, pp. 469–487. Palgrave Macmillan, 2018.

30. Banaji, Mahzarin R., and Anthony G. Greenwald. *Blindspot: Hidden Biases of Good People*. Bantam, 2016.

31. Levin, David Michael, ed. *Modernity and the Hegemony of Vision*. University of California Press, 1993.

32. Payne, B. Keith, and Bertram Gawronski. "A History of Implicit Social Cognition: Where Is It Coming From? Where Is It Now? Where Is It Going?" *Handbook of Implicit Social Cognition: Measurement, Theory, and Applications* 1 (2010): 1–15.

33. James, Robin. "Oppression, Privilege, & Aesthetics: The Use of the Aesthetic in Theories of Race, Gender, and Sexuality, and the Role of Race, Gender, and Sexuality in Philosophical Aesthetics." *Philosophy Compass* 8, no. 2 (2013):104.

34. Molden, Daniel C. "Understanding Priming Effects in Social Psychology: What Is 'Social Priming' and How Does It Occur?" *Social Cognition* 32, Supplement (2014): 1–11.

35. Sensoy, Özlem, and Robin DiAngelo. *Is Everyone Really Equal? An Introduction to Key Concepts in Social Justice Education*. Teachers College Press, 2012.

36. Menakem, Resmaa. *My Grandmother's Hands: Racialized Trauma and the Pathway to Mending Our Hearts and Bodies*. Central Recovery Press, 2017, 245.

37. Menakem, Resmaa. *My Grandmother's Hands: Racialized Trauma and the Pathway to Mending Our Hearts and Bodies*, 245.

38. Wilkerson, Isabel. *Caste: The Origins of Our Discontents*. Random House, 2020.

39. Menakem, Resmaa. *Grandmother's Hands: Racialized Trauma and the Pathway to Mending Our Hearts and Bodies*, xx.

40. Banaji, Mahzarin R., and Anthony G. Greenwald. *Blindspot: Hidden Biases of Good People*.

41. Banaji, Mahzarin R., and Anthony G. Greenwald. *Blindspot: Hidden Biases of Good People*, 69.

42. Nickerson, Raymond S. "Confirmation Bias: A Ubiquitous Phenomenon in Many Guises." *Review of General Psychology* 2, no. 2 (1998): 175–220.

43. Banaji, Mahzarin R., and Anthony G. Greenwald. *Blindspot: Hidden Biases of Good People*, 105.

44. Wilkerson, Isabel. *Caste: The Origins of Our Discontents*.

45. Wilkerson, Isabel. *Caste: The Origins of Our Discontents*, 304.

46. Payne and Gawronski. "A History of Implicit Social Cognition: Where Is It Coming From? Where Is It Now? Where Is It Going?" *Handbook of Implicit Social Cognition: Measurement, Theory, and Applications*.

47. Shotwell, Alexis. "Shame in Alterities: Adrian Piper, Intersubjectivity, and the Racial Formation of Identity." In *The Shock of the Other*, pp. 127–136. Brill, 2007.

48. Ahmed, Sara. *On Being Included: Racism and Diversity in Institutional Life*. Duke University Press, 2012.

49. Tomiyama, A. Janet, Deborah Carr, Ellen M. Granberg, Brenda Major, Eric Robinson, Angelina R. Sutin, and Alexandra Brewis. "How and Why Weight Stigma Drives the Obesity 'Epidemic' and Harms Health." *BMC Medicine* 16, no. 1 (2018): 1–6; Schwartz, Marlene B., Lenny R. Vartanian, Brian A. Nosek, and Kelly D. Brownell. "The Influence of One's Own Body Weight on Implicit and Explicit Anti-Fat Bias." *Obesity* 14, no. 3 (2006): 440–447; Pierce, Edgar F., and Myra L. Daleng. "Distortion of Body Image Among Elite Female Dancers." *Perceptual and Motor Skills* 87, no. 3 (1998): 769–770.

50. Kuppers, Petra. "Accessible Education: Aesthetics, Bodies and Disability." *Research in Dance Education* 1, no. 2 (2000): 119–131; Aujla, Imogen J., and Emma Redding. "Barriers to Dance Training for Young People with Disabilities." *British Journal of Special Education* 40, no. 2 (2013): 80–85; Hall, Joshua

M. "Philosophy of Dance and Disability." *Philosophy Compass* 13, no. 12 (2018): e12551.
  51. Mengel, Friederike, Jan Sauermann, and Ulf Zölitz. "Gender Bias in Teaching Evaluations." *Journal of the European Economic Association* 17, no. 2 (2019): 535–566; Bennett, Sheila K. "Student Perceptions of and Expectations for Male and Female Instructors: Evidence Relating to the Question of Gender Bias in Teaching Evaluation." *Journal of Educational Psychology* 74, no. 2 (1982): 170.

Chapter 1

  1. I have sourced and integrated and overlapped both Robin DiAngelo's article and Sheri Schmit's work in explaining the cycle of oppression for the Cycle of Oppression section. The terms defined in this explanation of the cycle of oppression are referring to their definitions specifically in a social justice context.
  2. DiAngelo, Robin. "THE CYCLE OF OPPRESSION." *Counterpoints* 497 (2016): 83–95.
  3. DiAngelo, Robin. "THE CYCLE OF OPPRESSION," and Schmidt, Sheri Lyn. "Cycle of Oppression," http://www.uas.alaska.edu/juneau/activities/safezone/docs/cycle_oppression.pdf (accessed May 29, 2018).
  4. Schmidt, "Cycle of Oppression," 1.
  5. This system of organizing and analyzing aspects of human movement was originally created by Rudolf Laban and will be discussed in further detail later in the book.
  6. Sensoy, Özlem, and Robin DiAngelo. *Is Everyone Really Equal? An Introduction to Key Concepts in Social Justice Education*, 32.
  7. Schmidt, Sheri. "Cycle of Oppression," 1.
  8. Davis, Crystal U., and Jesse Phillips-Fein. "Tendus and Tenancy: Black Dancers and the White Landscape of Dance Education." In *The Palgrave Handbook of Race and the Arts in Education*, pp. 571–584. Palgrave Macmillan, 2018.
  9. Schupp, Karen. "Dance Competition Culture and Commercial Dance: Intertwined Aesthetics, Values, and practices." *Journal of Dance Education* 19, no. 2 (2019): 58–67; Vincent, Christian John-Devi. "Bridging the Gap: Between Commercial Dance and Dance in Higher Education." PhD diss., UC Irvine, 2015.
  10. Davis, Crystal U., and Jesse Phillips-Fein. "Tendus and Tenancy: Black Dancers and the White Landscape of Dance Education." In *The Palgrave Handbook of Race and the Arts in Education*, pp. 571–584. Palgrave Macmillan, 2018.
  11. DiAngelo, Robin. "THE CYCLE OF OPPRESSION," 87.
  12. James, Robin. "Oppression, Privilege, & Aesthetics: The Use of the Aesthetic in Theories of Race, Gender, and Sexuality, and the Role of Race, Gender, and Sexuality in Philosophical Aesthetics," 102.
  13. James, Robin. "Oppression, Privilege, & Aesthetics: The Use of the Aesthetic in Theories of Race, Gender, and Sexuality, and the Role of Race, Gender, and Sexuality in Philosophical Aesthetics."
  14. James, Robin. "Oppression, Privilege, & Aesthetics: The Use of the Aesthetic in Theories of Race, Gender, and Sexuality, and the Role of Race, Gender, and Sexuality in Philosophical Aesthetic," 113.
  15. Jackson, Philip Wesley. *Life in Classrooms*. Teachers College Press, 1990; Stinson, Susan W. "The Hidden Curriculum of Gender in Dance Education." *Journal of Dance Education* 5, no. 2 (2005): 51–57; Yakhlef, Ali. "The Corporeality of Practice-Based Learning." *Organization Studies* 31, no. 4 (2010): 409–430.
  16. Macedonia, Manuela. "Embodied Learning: Why at School the Mind Needs the Body." *Frontiers in Psychology* 10 (2019): 2098.
  17. Davis, Crystal U., and Jesse Phillips-Fein. "Tendus and Tenancy: Black Dancers and the White Landscape of Dance Education."
  18. DiAngelo, Robin. *White Fragility: Why It's So Hard for White People to Talk About Racism*. Beacon Press, 2018, 42.
  19. Apfelbaum, Evan P., Kristin Pauker, Nalini Ambady, Samuel R. Sommers, and Michael I. Norton. "Learning (Not) to Talk about Race: When Older Children Underperform in Social Categorization." *Developmental Psychology* 44, no. 5 (2008): 1513; Martin, Carol Lynn, and Diane Ruble. "Children's Search for Gender Cues: Cognitive Perspectives on Gender Development." *Current Directions in Psychological Science* 13, no. 2 (2004): 67–70.
  20. Moore and Yamamoto. *Beyond*

Words: Movement Observation and Analysis, 52.
21. Sue, Derald Wing. *Microaggressions in Everyday Life: Race, Gender, and Sexual Orientation.* John Wiley & Sons, 2010, 5.
22. James, Robin. "Oppression, Privilege, & Aesthetics: The Use of the Aesthetic in Theories of Race, Gender, and Sexuality, and the Role of Race, Gender, and Sexuality in Philosophical Aesthetics."
23. Bates, Thomas R. "Gramsci and the Theory of Hegemony." *Journal of the History of Ideas* 36, no. 2 (1975): 351–366.
24. Davis, Crystal U., and Jesse Phillips-Fein. "Tendus and Tenancy: Black Dancers and the White Landscape of Dance Education."
25. Hancock, Black Hawk. "4. STEPPIN' OUT OF WHITENESS." In *American Allegory*, pp. 161–194. University of Chicago Press, 2013.

Chapter 2

1. "Project Implicit." https://implicit.harvard.edu/implicit/takeatest.html (Accessed April 29, 2018).
2. Cikara, Mina, Emile G. Bruneau, and Rebecca R. Saxe. "Us and Them: Intergroup Failures of Empathy." *Current Directions in Psychological Science* 20, no. 3 (2011): 149–153.
3. O'Brien, Kerry S., John A. Hunter, and Mike Banks. "Implicit Anti-Fat Bias in Physical Educators: Physical Attributes, Ideology and Socialization." *International Journal of Obesity* 31, no. 2 (2007): 309.
4. Additional published research that supports this finding include Tajfel and Turner; Guimond; Sechrist & Stangor; Dambrun et al.; Guimond & Palmer; O'Brien, Kerry S., John A. Hunter, and Mike Banks. "Implicit Anti-Fat Bias in Physical Educators: Physical Attributes, Ideology and Socialization."
5. Hudson, Sa-kiera Tiarra Jolynn, Mina Cikara, and Jim Sidanius. "Preference for Hierarchy Is Associated with Reduced Empathy and Increased Counter-Empathy Towards Others, Especially Out-Group Targets." *Journal of Experimental Social Psychology* 85 (2019): 103871.
6. Kant, Immanuel. *Observations on the Feeling of the Beautiful and Sublime.* University of California Press, 2003.
7. Banaji, Mahzarin R., Max H. Bazerman, and Dolly Chugh. "How (Un)ethical Are You?" *Harvard Business Review* (Dec. 2003), 3–10.
8. Banaji, Bazerman, and Chugh. "How (Un)ethical Are You?"
9. Vai, Isabelle. Dance Data Project. July 2020. https://www.dancedataproject.com/research/ (accessed April 23, 2020).
10. Davis, Crystal U. "Laying New Ground: Uprooting White Privilege and Planting Seeds of Equity and Inclusivity." In *Dance Education and Responsible Citizenship: Promoting Civic Engagement Through Effective Dance Pedagogies*, pp. 58–70. Routledge, 2019.
11. Smith, Phillip A. "Does Racism Exist in the Hiring and Promotion of K-12 School Administrators?" *Urban Education Research & Policy Annuals* 4, no. 1 (2016): 122–136; Isaac, Carol, Barbara Lee, and Molly Carnes. "Interventions That Affect Gender Bias in Hiring: A Systematic Review." *Academic Medicine: Journal of the Association of American Medical Colleges* 84, no. 10 (2009): 1440; O'Meara, KerryAnn, Dawn Culpepper, and Lindsey L. Templeton. "Nudging Toward Diversity: Applying Behavioral Design to Faculty Hiring." *Review of Educational Research* 90, no. 3 (2020): 311–348; Sanchez, Jafeth E., and Bill Thornton. "Gender Issues in K-12 Educational Leadership." *Advancing Women in Leadership Journal* 30 (2010).
12. Aronson, Brittany A. "The White Savior Industrial Complex: A Cultural Studies Analysis of a Teacher Educator, Savior Film, and Future Teachers." *Journal of Critical Thought and Praxis* 6, no. 3 (2017): ar3.

Chapter 3

1. James, Robin. "Oppression, Privilege, & Aesthetics: The Use of the Aesthetic in Theories of Race, Gender, and Sexuality, and the Role of Race, Gender, and Sexuality in Philosophical Aesthetics."
2. McCarthy-Brown, Nyama. "Owners of Dance: How Dance Is Controlled and Whitewashed in the Teaching of Dance Forms." In *The Palgrave Handbook of Race and the Arts in Education*, pp. 469–487. Palgrave Macmillan, 2018.

3. James, Robin. "Oppression, Privilege, & Aesthetics: The Use of the Aesthetic in Theories of Race, Gender, and Sexuality, and the Role of Race, Gender, and Sexuality in Philosophical Aesthetics"; Kant, Immanuel. *Observations on the Feeling of the Beautiful and Sublime*.

4. Schupp, Karen, and Nyama McCarthy-Brown. "Dancing with Diversity: Students' Perceptions of Diversity in Postsecondary Dance Programs" (2018).

5. James, Robin. " Oppression, Privilege, & Aesthetics: The Use of the Aesthetic in Theories of Race, Gender, and Sexuality, and the Role of Race, Gender, and Sexuality in Philosophical Aesthetics," 108.

6. Menakem, Resmaa. *My Grandmother's Hands: Racialized Trauma and the Pathway to Mending Our Hearts and Bodies*.

7. Menakem, Resmaa. *My Grandmother's Hands: Racialized Trauma and the Pathway to Mending Our Hearts and Bodies*, 6.

8. Menakem, Resmaa. *My Grandmother's Hands: Racialized Trauma and the Pathway to Mending Our Hearts and Bodies*, 4.

9. Menakem, Resmaa. *My Grandmother's Hands: Racialized Trauma and the Pathway to Mending Our Hearts and Bodies*, 6.

10. "Project Implicit." https://implicit.harvard.edu/implicit/takeatest.html (Accessed April 29, 2018).

11. DiAngelo, Robin. *White Fragility: Why It's So Hard for White People to Talk about Racism*, 50.

12. Mills, Charles. "White Ignorance." *Race and Epistemologies of Ignorance* 247 (2007): 26–31.

13. Cohen, Stanley. *States of Denial: Knowing about Atrocities and Suffering*. John Wiley & Sons, 2001.

14. Banaji, Mahzarin R., Max H. Bazerman, and Dolly Chugh. "How (Un)ethical Are You?" *Harvard Business Review* (2003), 4.

15. Monroe, Raquel L. "'I Don't Want to do African … What About My Technique?': Transforming Dancing Places into Spaces in the Academy." *Journal of Pan African Studies* 4, no. 6 (2011): 38.

16. Eberhardt, Jennifer L. *Biased: Uncovering the Hidden Prejudice That Shapes What We See, Think, and Do*. Penguin, 2020.

17. Gn 1:26.

18. Blakey, Michael L. "Man and Nature, White and Other." *Decolonizing Anthropology* (1991): 15–23.

19. DiAngelo, Robin. *White Fragility: Why It's So Hard for White People to Talk about Racism*.

20. There was an African princess project under development in 2018 and due to hit theaters in 2021. Further context on the history of African and African American princesses can be seen in this article: https://www.nbcnews.com/news/nbcblk/disney-s-picks-live-action-fairytale-about-young-african-princess-n895421]; Eberhardt also discusses evidence of this association of Black people with ape being pervasive even for people who attest to having no conscious awareness of the association.

21. Eberhardt, Jennifer L. *Biased: Uncovering the Hidden Prejudice That Shapes What We See, Think, and Do*. Penguin, 2020.

22. Cikara, Mina, Emile G. Bruneau, and Rebecca R. Saxe. "Us and Them: Intergroup Failures of Empathy." *Current Directions in Psychological Science* 20, no. 3 (2011): 149–153.

23. Cikara, Mina, Emile G. Bruneau, and Rebecca R. Saxe. "Us and Them: Intergroup Failures of Empathy." *Current Directions in Psychological Science* 20, no. 3 (2011): 149–153.

24. Moore, Carol-Lynne, and Kaoru Yamamoto. *Beyond Words: Movement Observation and Analysis*.

25. Moore, Carol-Lynne, and Kaoru Yamamoto. *Beyond Words: Movement Observation and Analysis*, 47.

26. Moore, Carol-Lynne, and Kaoru Yamamoto. *Beyond Words: Movement Observation and Analysis*.

27. Eberhardt, Jennifer L. *Biased: Uncovering the Hidden Prejudice That Shapes What We See, Think, and Do*.

28. Harris, Lasana T., and Susan T. Fiske. "Dehumanizing the Lowest of the Low: Neuroimaging Responses to Extreme Out-Groups." *Psychological Science* 17, no. 10 (2006): 847–853.

Chapter 4

1. Levinson, Justin D. "Forgotten Racial Equality: Implicit Bias,

Decisionmaking, and Misremembering." *Duke LJ* 57 (2007): 345, 423.

2. Moore, Carol-Lynne, and Kaoru Yamamoto. *Beyond Words: Movement Observation and Analysis*. Routledge, 2012, 54–55.

3. The acronym LGBTQ stands for lesbian, gay, bisexual, transgender, and queer.

4. Mills, Charles. "White Ignorance." *Race and Epistemologies of Ignorance* 247 (2007): 26–31.

5. For further information on somatic reflective processes, see *My Grandmother's Hands: Racialized Trauma and the Pathway to Mending our Hearts and Bodies* (2017) by Resmaa Menakem.

6. Bardet, Marie, and Florencio Noceti. "With Descartes, Against Dualism." *Journal of Dance & Somatic Practices* 4, no. 2 (2012): 195–209.

7. Essed, Philomena, and David Theo Goldberg. "Cloning Cultures: The Social Injustices of Sameness." *Ethnic and Racial Studies* 25, no. 6 (2002): 1067.

8. https://www.dancedataproject.com/wp-content/uploads/2020/08/July-2020-Season-Report.pdf.

9. https://datausa.io/profile/soc/dancers-choreographers#demographics.

10. Levinson, Justin D. "Forgotten Racial Equality: Implicit Bias, Decisionmaking, and Misremembering." *Duke LJ* 57 (2007): 345.

11. Davis, Crystal U., and Jesse Phillips-Fein. "Tendus and Tenancy: Black Dancers and the White Landscape of Dance Education." In *The Palgrave Handbook of Race and the Arts in Education*, pp. 571–584. Palgrave Macmillan, 2018.

12. DiAngelo, Robin. *White Fragility: Why It's So Hard for White People to Talk about Racism*. Beacon Press, 2018.

13. Sue, Derald Wing. (2010). *Microaggressions in Everyday Life: Race, Gender, and Sexual Orientation*.

14. Sue, Derald Wing, Christina M. Capodilupo, Gina C. Torino, Jennifer M. Bucceri, Aisha Holder, Kevin L. Nadal, and Marta Esquilin. "Racial Microaggressions in Everyday Life: Implications for Clinical Practice." *American Psychologist* 62, no. 4 (2007): 271.

15. Moore and Yamamoto. *Beyond Words: Movement Observation and Analysis*.

16. Moore and Yamamoto. *Beyond Words: Movement Observation and Analysis*, 52.

17. Wahl, Colleen. *Laban/Bartenieff Movement Studies: Contemporary Applications*. Human Kinetics, 2019.

18. Fernandes, Ciane. *The Moving Researcher: Laban/Bartenieff Movement Analysis in Performing Arts Education and Creative Arts Therapies*. Jessica Kingsley, 2014.

19. I myself certified as a Laban-Bartenieff Movement Analyst (CLMA) through the Integrated Movement Studies program, certified at the intermediate level of Labanotation, and have taken workshops in the Language of Dance, a system based on Laban's work and further developed by Dr. Ann Hutchinson Guest.

20. Bradley, Karen K. *Rudolf Laban*. Routledge, 2018.

21. Labanotation is one of the many systems of movement analysis, theory, and documentation that have blossomed from the work of Laban. It is a notation system based on the work of Rudolf Laban for documenting human movement with a great deal of accuracy and detail.

22. Bartenieff, Irmgard, Peggy Hackney, Betty True Jones, Judy Van Zile, and Carl Wolz. "The Potential of Movement Analysis as a Research Tool: A Preliminary Analysis." *Dance Research Journal* 16, no. 1 (1984): 3.

23. Bartenieff, et al. "The Potential of Movement Analysis as a Research Tool: A Preliminary Analysis."

24. Farnell, Brenda. "It Goes Without Saying—but Not Always." In *Dance in the Field*, pp. 145–160. Palgrave Macmillan, 1999.

25. I open the discussion here beyond the two systems I am certified in, LBMA and Labanotation, to a broader reach of Laban-oriented systems of movement analysis, documentation, and principles used in dance education including systems like Language of Dance (LOD) developed by Dr. Hutchinson Guest.

26. Farnell makes clear the value of Labanotation in her example of illustrating one action-sign three different ways: "i) hand moves away from chest; ii) hand moves forward; iii) 'ethno-graph'—hand moves toward east" (p. 156). She explains in the Assiniboine story that is the source of this movement, the only accurate action-sign is the third example.

27. Davis, Crystal U., and Jesse Phillips-Fein. "Tendus and Tenancy: Black Dancers and the White Landscape of Dance Education."
28. Rasmussen, Birgit Brander, Eric Klinenberg, Irene J. Nexica, and Matt Wray, eds. *The Making and Unmaking of Whiteness*. Duke University Press, 2001.
29. Banerji, Anurima. "The Laws of Movement: The Natyashastra as Archive for Indian Classical Dance." *Contemporary Theatre Review* 31, no. 1–2 (2021): 132–152.
30. Moore and Yamamoto. *Beyond Words: Movement Observation and Analysis*.
31. Note that the term "blind spot" used by Banaji and Greenwald in and of itself reflects an able-bodied bias toward seeing; Banaji, Mahzarin R., and Anthony G. Greenwald. *Blindspot: Hidden Biases of Good People*.
32. Holroyd, Jules, and Katherine Puddifoot. "6. Epistemic Injustice and Implicit Bias." *An Introduction to Implicit Bias: Knowledge, Justice, and the Social Mind* (2020).
33. Holroyd, Jules, and Katherine Puddifoot. "6. Epistemic Injustice and Implicit Bias."
34. Noble, Safiya Umoja. *Algorithms of Oppression: How Search Engines Reinforce Racism*. NYU Press, 2018.

Chapter 5

1. Levinson, Justin D. "Forgotten Racial Equality: Implicit Bias, Decisionmaking, and Misremembering." *Duke LJ* 57 (2007): 345.
2. Levinson. "Forgotten Facial Equality: Implicit Bias, Decisionmaking, and Misremembering," 379.
3. Payne, B. Keith, and Bertram Gawronski. "A History of Implicit Social Cognition: Where Is It Coming From? Where Is It Now? Where Is It Going?" *Handbook of Implicit Social Cognition: Measurement, Theory, and Applications* 1 (2010): 1–15.
4. This flower and bug example is taken from a sample IAT provided in the following reference: Banaji, Mahzarin R., and Anthony G. Greenwald. *Blindspot: Hidden Biases of Good People*. Bantam, 2016.
5. The Glossary of Education Reform, s.v. "hidden curriculum," https://www.edglossary.org/hidden-curriculum/#:~:text=Hidden%20curriculum%20refers%20to%20the,that%20students%20learn%20in%20school.&text=Cultural%20expectations%3A%20The%20academic%2C%20social,educators%20communicate%20messages%20to%20students.
6. Banaji, Mahzarin R., Max H. Bazerman, and Dolly Chugh. "How (Un)ethical Are You?" *Harvard Business Review* (Dec. 2003), 3–10.
7. Harris, Michael M., Filip Lievens, and Greet Van Hoye. "'I think they discriminated against me': Using Prototype Theory and Organizational Justice Theory for Understanding Perceived Discrimination in Selection and Promotion Situations." *International Journal of Selection and Assessment* 12, no. 1-2 (2004): 54.
8. Banaji, Mahzarin R., and Anthony G. Greenwald. *Blindspot: Hidden Biases of Good People*.
9. Banaji, Mahzarin R., and Anthony G. Greenwald. *Blindspot: Hidden Biases of Good People*.
10. Gladwell, Malcolm. *Blink: The Power of Thinking Without Thinking*. Little, Brown, 2005.
11. Banaji, Mahzarin R., and Anthony G. Greenwald. *Blindspot: Hidden Biases of Good People*.
12. Eberhardt, Jennifer L. *Biased: Uncovering the Hidden Prejudice That Shapes What We See, Think, and Do*. Penguin, 2020.
13. Allport, Gordon Willard, Kenneth Clark, and Thomas Pettigrew. *The Nature of Prejudice (25th Anniversary Edition)*. Basic Books, 1979.
14. Moore and Yamamoto. *Beyond Words: Movement Observation and Analysis*.
15. Moore and Yamamoto. *Beyond Words: Movement Observation and Analysis*, 54.
16. Moore and Yamamoto. *Beyond Words: Movement Observation and Analysis*.
17. Holroyd, Jules, and Katherine Puddifoot. "Epistemic Injustice and Implicit Bias." In *An Introduction to Implicit Bias*, pp. 116–133. Routledge, 2020.
18. Ahmed, Sara. *On Being Included: Racism and Diversity in Institutional Life*. Duke University Press, 2012.

19. Green, Jill. "Moving In, Out, Through, and Beyond the Tensions Between Experience and Social Construction in Somatic Theory." *Journal of Dance & Somatic Practices* 7, no. 1 (2015): 7–19.
20. Eddy, Martha. "Somatic Practices and Dance: Global Influences." *Dance Research Journal* 34, no. 2 (2002): 46–62.
21. Johnson, Don Hanlon, ed. *Diverse Bodies, Diverse Practices: Toward an Inclusive Somatics.* North Atlantic Books, 2018.
22. Bell, Karine. Rooted Global Village. https://www.rootedandembodied.com/. Accessed June 26, 2021.

Chapter 6

1. Holroyd, Jules, Robin Scaife, and Tom Stafford. "Responsibility for Implicit Bias." *Philosophy Compass* 12, no. 3 (2017): e12410.
2. Banaji, Mahzarin R., and Anthony G. Greenwald. *Blindspot: Hidden Biases of Good People.* Bantam, 2016.
3. Holroyd, Jules, Robin Scaife, and Tom Stafford. "Responsibility for Implicit Bias." *Philosophy Compass* 12, no. 3 (2017): e12410.
4. https://implicit.harvard.edu/implicit/takeatest.html.
5. Banaji, Mahzarin R., "Implicit Bias in the Mind and in the Classroom," presentation at the National Assn. of Independent Schools People of Color Conf., Dec. 4, 2015, Tampa, FL.
6. This term is how Banaji and Greenwald (2016) refer to the cognitive effects of implicit bias in their book, *Blindspot: Hidden Biases of Good People.*
7. McCarthy-Brown, Nyama. *Dance Pedagogy for a Diverse World: Culturally Relevant Teaching in Theory, Research and Practice.* McFarland, 2017.
8. Bartenieff, Irmgard, and Forrestine Paulay. "Cross-Cultural Study of Dance: Description and Implications." Undated. Q1-1-1 to Q3-4-3, Box R/S 18, Folder 10. *Irmgard Bartenieff Papers.* Special Collections in Performing Arts, Michelle Smith Performing Arts Library, Clarice Smith Performing Arts Center, University of Maryland, College Park, MD.
9. Lerman, Liz, and John Borstel. *Liz Lerman's Critical Response Process: A Method for Getting Useful Feedback on Anything You Make, From Dance to Dessert.* Liz Lerman Dance Exchange, 2003.
10. Freire, Paulo. *Pedagogy of Freedom: Ethics, Democracy, and Civic Courage.* Rowman & Littlefield, 2000.
11. Banaji and Greenwald. *Blindspot: Hidden Biases of Good People*; Moore and Yamamoto. *Beyond Words: Movement Observation and Analysis.*
12. McCarthy-Brown, Nyama. *Dance Pedagogy for a Diverse World: Culturally Relevant Teaching in Theory, Research and Practice.* McFarland, 2017.
13. Taylor, Charles. "The Politics of Recognition." *New Contexts of Canadian Criticism* 98 (1997): 25–73.
14. Kerr-Berry, Julie. "Counterstorytelling in Concert Dance History Pedagogy: Challenging the White Dancing Body." In *The Palgrave Handbook of Race and the Arts in Education*, pp. 137–155. Palgrave Macmillan, 2018; Whatley, Sarah. "The Spectacle of Difference: Dance and Disability on Screen." *The International Journal of Screendance* 1 (2018).
15. Eberhardt. *Biased: Uncovering the Hidden Prejudice That Shapes What We See, Think, and Do.*
16. Eberhardt. *Biased: Uncovering the Hidden Prejudice That Shapes What We See, Think, and Do,* 125.
17. Eberhardt. *Biased: Uncovering the Hidden Prejudice That Shapes What We See, Think, and Do,* 125.
18. Eberhardt. *Biased: Uncovering the Hidden Prejudice That Shapes What We See, Think, and Do,* 125.
19. For more on knowledge and community practices that are born from collective sharing and exchange, I recommend Brown, Adrienne M. *Emergent Strategy: Shaping Change, Changing Worlds.* AK Press, 2017.
20. Greene, Maxine. "Diversity and Inclusion: Toward a Curriculum for Human Beings." *Teachers College Record* 95, no. 2 (1993): 211–221.
21. Adrienne M. Brown speaks of this in her book, *Emergent Strategy: Shaping Change, Changing Worlds* (2017). Tyson Yunkaporta also speaks of this in his book, *Sand Talk: How Indigenous Thinking Can Save the World* (2017).
22. Greene. "Diversity and Inclusion: Toward a Curriculum for Human Beings," 212–213.
23. Greene. "Diversity and Inclusion:

Toward a Curriculum for Human Beings," 220.

24. Gibbons, Elizabeth. *Teaching Dance: The Spectrum of Styles.* AuthorHouse, 2007.

25. Gibbons, Elizabeth. *Teaching Dance: The Spectrum of Styles,* p. v.

26. Gibbons, Elizabeth. *Teaching Dance: The Spectrum of Styles,* p. v.

27. Moore and Yamamoto. *Beyond Words: Movement Observation and Analysis,* 46.

28. Storey, Valerie A., and Victor CX Wang. "Critical Friends Protocol: Andragogy and Learning in a Graduate Classroom." *Adult Learning* 28, no. 3 (2017): 107–114; Burke, Wendy, Gary E. Marx, and James E. Berry. "Maintaining, Reframing, and Disrupting Traditional Expectations and Outcomes for Professional Development with Critical Friends Groups." *The Teacher Educator* 46, no. 1 (2010): 32–52.

29. Storey, Valerie A., and Victor CX Wang. "Critical Friends Protocol: Andragogy and Learning in a Graduate Classroom." *Adult Learning* 28, no. 3 (2017): 107–114.

30. Wernick, Laura J., Michael R. Woodford, and Alex Kulick. "LGBTQQ Youth Using Participatory Action Research and Theater to Effect Change: Moving Adult Decision-Makers to Create Youth-Centered Change." *Journal of Community Practice* 22, no. 1–2 (2014): 47–66.

31. In Wernick, Woodford, and Kulick's article, this acronym stands for lesbian, gay, bisexual, transgender, queer, and questioning. Thus, I will use this term when discussing the research shared in this article.

32. Boal, Augusto. *Theater of the Oppressed.* Pluto Press, 2000.

33. Farnell, Brenda. "It Goes Without Saying—but Not Always." In *Dance in the Field,* pp. 145–160. Palgrave Macmillan, 1999.

34. Menakem, Resmaa. *My Grandmother's Hands: Racialized Trauma and the Pathway to Mending Our Hearts and Bodies,* 168.

35. Menakem, Resmaa. *My Grandmother's Hands: Racialized Trauma and the Pathway to Mending Our Hearts and Bodies..*

36. Singleton, Glenn E. *Courageous Conversations About Race: A Field Guide for Achieving Equity in Schools.* Corwin Press, 2014; Pinkus, Ari. "After the People of Color Conference...," National Assn. of Independent Schools People of Color Conference, Dec. 9, 2015, https://www.nais.org/learn/independent-ideas/december-2015/after-the-people-of-color-conference,-10-guidepost/.

Chapter 7

1. See Appendix C for my starting set of community norms.

2. Charlton, James I. *Nothing About Us Without Us.* University of California Press, 1998.

3. Arnold, Rick. *Educating for a Change.* Doris Marshall Institute, Toronto, 1991; Just Associates and We Rise. "Flower Power: Our Intersecting Identities." https://werise-toolkit.org/en/system/tdf/pdf/tools/Power-Flower-Our-Intersecting-Identities_0.pdf?file=1&force=#:~:text=get%20the%20concept.-,The%20central%20part%20of%20the%20flower%20represents%20a%20person's%20nationality,%3A%20male%3B%20religion%3A%20Catholic. Accessed June 26, 2021.

4. Montgomery, Mary Lynn, and Mary Jetter. "'I am from' Activity Guide: A Tool to Foster Student Interaction in the Classroom." Global Programs and Strategy Alliance at the University of Minnesota, 2016. https://global.umn.edu/icc/documents/I_Am_From_Faculty_Guide.pdf. Accessed May 8, 2021.

5. Guest, Ann Hutchinson. *Choreo-Graphics: A Comparison of Dance Notation Systems from the Fifteenth Century to the Present.* Psychology Press, 1998.

6. Lerman, Liz, and John Borstel. *Liz Lerman's Critical Response Process: A Method for Getting Useful Feedback on Anything You Make, From Dance to Dessert.* Liz Lerman Dance Exchange, 2003.

7. Clemente, Karen. "Bylines and Bias Part II." In *National Dance Education Organization: Speaking with Our Feet: Advocating, Analyzing, and Advancing Dance Education.* Washington, D.C., October 6–10, 2016.

8. See discussion and references (Fentroy, Howard, Spears, Williams) from Introduction.

9. Clemente, Karen. "Modern Dance

History" (syllabus, Ursinus College, Collegeville, PA, 2019).
10. Clemente. "Modern Dance History."
11. Clemente. "Modern Dance History."
12. See Appendix B for a fuller outline of this curriculum.
13. Lepecki, André. *Of the Presence of the Body: Essays on Dance and Performance Theory*, Wesleyan University Press, 2004.
14. Allen, B.J., and M.P. Orbe. "Race Matters." *Journal of Applied Communication Research* 19 (2008): 201–220.
15. Freire, Paulo. *Pedagogy of Freedom: Ethics, Democracy, and Civic Courage*. Rowman & Littlefield, 2000.
16. Arao, Brian, and Kristi Clemens. "From Safe Spaces to Brave Spaces." *The Art of Effective Facilitation: Reflections from Social Justice Educators* (2013): 135–150.
17. Sensoy, Özlem, and Robin DiAngelo. *Is Everyone Really Equal? An Introduction to Key Concepts in Social Justice Education*. Teachers College Press, 2012.
18. Shapiro, Sherry B. *Dance, Power, and Difference: Critical and Feminist Perspectives on Dance Education*. Human Kinetics, 1998, 1.
19. Preston-Dunlop, Valerie, and Ana Sanchez-Colberg. *Dance and the Performative: A Choreological Perspective—Laban and Beyond*. Verve Publishing, 2002.
20. To see more information about this structure, access The Field's web page on Fieldwork, https://www.thefield.org/programs/fieldwork.
21. Lerman and Borstel. *Liz Lerman's Critical Response Process: A Method for Getting Useful Feedback on Anything You Make, From Dance to Dessert*.

Appendix B

1. Most of the norms are from the National Association of Independent Schools Student Diversity Leadership Conference (NAIS SDLC) statement.
2. Singleton, Glenn E. *Courageous Conversations About Race: A Field Guide for Achieving Equity in Schools*. Corwin Press, 2014.
3. Singleton, Glenn E. *Courageous Conversations About Race: A Field Guide for Achieving Equity in Schools*.

Works Cited

Adelstein, Janna, and Alicia Bannon. "State Supreme Court Diversity—April 2021 Update." Brennan Center for Justice, April 20, 2021, https://www.brennancenter.org/our-work/research-reports/state-supreme-court-diversity-april-2021-update.
Ahmed, Sara. *On Being Included: Racism and Diversity in Institutional Life*. Duke University Press, 2012.
Ahmed, Sara. "Racialized Bodies." In *Real Bodies*, pp. 46–63. Palgrave, 2002.
Airhihenbuwa, Collins O. "From 1619 to COVID-19: A double pandemic." *Health Promotion Practice* 21, no. 6 (2020): 857–858.
Allen, B.J., and M.P. Orbe. "Race Matters." *Journal of Applied Communication Research* 19 (2008): 201–220.
Allport, Gordon Willard, Kenneth Clark, and Thomas Pettigrew. *The Nature of Prejudice (25th Anniversary Edition)*. Basic Books, 1979.
Apfelbaum, Evan P., Kristin Pauker, Nalini Ambady, Samuel R. Sommers, and Michael I. Norton. "Learning (Not) to Talk about Race: When Older Children Underperform in Social Categorization." *Developmental Psychology* 44, no. 5 (2008): 1513–1518.
Arao, Brian, and Kristi Clemens. "From Safe Spaces to Brave Spaces." *The Art of Effective Facilitation: Reflections from Social Justice Educators* (2013): 135–150.
Arnold, Rick. *Educating for a Change*. Doris Marshall Institute, Toronto, 1991.
Aronson, Brittany A. "The White Savior Industrial Complex: A Cultural Studies Analysis of a Teacher Educator, Savior Film, and Future Teachers." *Journal of Critical Thought and Praxis* 6, no. 3 (2017): ar3.
Aujla, Imogen J., and Emma Redding. "Barriers to Dance Training for Young People with Disabilities." *British Journal of Special Education* 40, no. 2 (2013): 80–85.
Banaji, Mahzarin R., "Implicit Bias in the Mind and in the Classroom," presentation at the National Assn. of Independent Schools People of Color Conf., Dec. 4, 2015, Tampa, FL.
Banaji, Mahzarin R., and Anthony G. Greenwald. *Blindspot: Hidden Biases of Good People*. Bantam, 2016.
Banaji, Mahzarin R., Max H. Bazerman, and Dolly Chugh. "How (Un)ethical Are You?" *Harvard Business Review* (Dec. 2003), 3–10.
Banerji, Anurima. "The Laws of Movement: The Natyashastra as Archive for Indian Classical Dance." *Contemporary Theatre Review* 31, no. 1–2 (2021): 132–152.
Bardet, Marie, and Florencio Noceti. "With Descartes, Against Dualism." *Journal of Dance & Somatic Practices* 4, no. 2 (2012): 195–209.
Bartenieff, Irmgard, and Forrestine Paulay. "Cross-Cultural Study of Dance: Description and Implications." Undated. Q1-1-1 to Q3-4-3, Box R/S 18, Folder 10. Irmgard Bartenieff Papers. Special Collections in Performing Arts, Michelle Smith Performing Arts Library, Clarice Smith Performing Arts Center, University of Maryland, College Park, MD.
Bartenieff, Irmgard, Peggy Hackney, Betty True Jones, Judy Van Zile, and Carl Wolz. "The Potential of Movement Analysis as a Research Tool: A Preliminary Analysis." *Dance Research Journal* 16, no. 1 (1984): 3–26.

Works Cited

Bates, Thomas R. "Gramsci and the Theory of Hegemony." *Journal of the History of Ideas* 36, no. 2 (1975): 351–366.
Beeghly, Erin, and Alex Madva, eds. *An Introduction to Implicit Bias: Knowledge, Justice, and the Social Mind.* Routledge, 2020.
Bell, Karine. Rooted Global Village. https://www.rootedandembodied.com/. Accessed June 26, 2021.
Bennett, Sheila K. "Student Perceptions of and Expectations for Male and Female Instructors: Evidence Relating to the Question of Gender Bias in Teaching Evaluation." *Journal of Educational Psychology* 74, no. 2 (1982): 170.
Blakey, Michael L. "Man and Nature, White and Other." In *Decolonizing Anthropology*, 15–23. American Anthropological Assn., 1991.
Blume, Libby Balter. "Embodied [by] Dance: Adolescent De/Constructions of Body, Sex and Gender in Physical Education." *Sex Education: Sexuality, Society and Learning* 3, no. 2 (2003): 95–103.
Boal, Augusto. *Theater of the Oppressed.* Pluto Press, 2000.
Bradley, Karen K. *Rudolf Laban.* Routledge, 2018.
Brown, Adrienne M. *Emergent Strategy: Shaping Change, Changing Worlds.* AK Press, 2017.
Brustad, Robert. "A Critical-Postmodern Perspective on Knowledge Development in Human Movement." *Critical Postmodernism in Human Movement, Physical Education, and Sport* (1997): 87–98.
Buckland, Theresa, ed. *Dance in the Field: Theory, Methods and Issues in Dance Ethnography.* Springer, 1999.
Burke, Wendy, Gary E. Marx, and James E. Berry. "Maintaining, Reframing, and Disrupting Traditional Expectations and Outcomes for Professional Development with Critical Friends Groups." *The Teacher Educator* 46, no. 1 (2010): 32–52.
Bushwackers, choreographed by Kim Tapp, toured Fall 2000–Fall 2001.
Carter, Julian B. *The Heart of Whiteness: Normal Sexuality and Race in America, 1880–1940.* Duke University Press, 2007.
Charlton, James I. *Nothing about Us Without Us.* University of California Press, 1998.
Cikara, Mina, Emile G. Bruneau, and Rebecca R. Saxe. "Us and Them: Intergroup Failures of Empathy." *Current Directions in Psychological Science* 20, no. 3 (2011): 149–153.
Clemente, Karen. "Bylines and Bias Part II." National Dance Education Organization: Speaking with our Feet: Advocating, Analyzing, and Advancing Dance Education. Washington, D.C. October 6–10, 2016.
Clemente, Karen. "Modern Dance History: Post-Modern Dance." Syllabus, Ursinus College, Collegeville, PA, 2019.
Cohen, Stanley. *States of Denial: Knowing about Atrocities and Suffering.* John Wiley & Sons, 2001.
Dambrun, Michaël, Serge Guimond, and Sandra Duarte. "The Impact of Hierarchy-Enhancing vs. Attenuating Academic Major on Stereotyping: The Mediating Role of Perceived Social Norm." *Current Research in Social Psychology* 7, no. 8 (2002): 114–136.
DataUSA: Optometrists. https://datausa.io/profile/soc/optometrists#demographics. Accessed January 4, 2021.
Davis, Crystal U. "Laying New Ground: Uprooting White Privilege and Planting Seeds of Equity and Inclusivity." In *Dance Education and Responsible Citizenship: Promoting Civic Engagement Through Effective Dance Pedagogies*, pp. 58–70. Routledge, 2019.
Davis, Crystal U., and Jesse Phillips-Fein. "Tendus and Tenancy: Black Dancers and the White Landscape of Dance Education." In *The Palgrave Handbook of Race and the Arts in Education*, pp. 571–584. Palgrave Macmillan, 2018.
DiAngelo, Robin. "THE CYCLE OF OPPRESSION." *Counterpoints* 497 (2016): 83–95.
DiAngelo, Robin. *White Fragility: Why It's So Hard for White People to Talk about Racism.* Beacon Press, 2018.
Eberhardt, Jennifer L. *Biased: Uncovering the Hidden Prejudice That Shapes What We See, Think, and Do.* Penguin, 2020.
Eddy, Martha. "Somatic Practices and Dance: Global Influences." *Dance Research Journal* 34, no. 2 (2002): 46–62.

Works Cited

Essed, Philomena, and David Theo Goldberg. "Cloning Cultures: The Social Injustices of Sameness." *Ethnic and Racial Studies* 25, no. 6 (2002): 1066–1082.

"Examining the Demographic Compositions of U.S. Circuit and District Courts." https://www.americanprogress.org/issues/courts/reports/2020/02/13/480112/examining-demographic-compositions-u-s-circuit-district-courts/. Accessed January 4, 2021.

Farnell, Brenda. "It Goes Without Saying—but Not Always." In *Dance in the Field*, pp. 145–160. Palgrave Macmillan, 1999.

Fentroy, Chyrstyn Mariah. "My Experience as a Black Ballerina in a World of Implicit Bias." *Pointe Magazine*, June 5, 2020. https://www.pointemagazine.com/chyrstyn-fentroy-2646155391.html (accessed December 4, 2020).

Fernandes, Ciane. *The Moving Researcher: Laban/Bartenieff Movement Analysis in Performing Arts Education and Creative Arts Therapies.* Jessica Kingsley, 2014.

Frankenberg, Ruth, ed. *Displacing Whiteness: Essays in Social and Cultural Criticism.* Duke University Press, 1997.

Freire, Paulo. *Pedagogy of Freedom: Ethics, Democracy, and Civic Courage.* Rowman & Littlefield, 2000.

Fricker, Miranda. *Epistemic Injustice: Power and the Ethics of Knowing.* Oxford University Press, 2007.

Gibbons, Elizabeth. *Teaching Dance: The Spectrum of Styles.* AuthorHouse, 2007.

Gladwell, Malcolm. *Blink: The Power of Thinking Without Thinking.* Little, Brown, 2005.

The Glossary of Education Reform, s.v. "hidden curriculum." https://www.edglossary.org. Accessed January 12, 2022.

Gottschild, Brenda. *The Black Dancing Body: A Geography from Coon to Cool.* Springer, 2016.

Grablick, Colleen. "Kennedy Center Receives $25 Million in Federal Relief, Furloughs NSO Members." March, 26, 2020. https://dcist.com/story/20/03/26/kennedy-center-receives-25-million-in-relief-bill-support-from-president-trump/. Accessed October 23, 2020.

Green, Jill. "Moving In, Out, Through, and Beyond the Tensions Between Experience and Social Construction in Somatic Theory." *Journal of Dance & Somatic Practices* 7, no. 1 (2015): 7–19.

Greene, Maxine. "Diversity and Inclusion: Toward a Curriculum for Human Beings." *Teachers College Record* 95, no. 2 (1993): 211–221.

Guest, Ann Hutchinson. *Choreo-Graphics: A Comparison of Dance Notation Systems from the Fifteenth Century to the Present.* Psychology Press, 1998.

Guimond, Serge. "Group Socialization and Prejudice: The Social Transmission of Intergroup Attitudes and Beliefs." *European Journal of Social Psychology* 30, no. 3 (2000): 335–354.

Guimond, Serge, and Douglas L. Palmer. "The Political Socialization of Commerce and Social Science Students: Epistemic Authority and Attitude Change 1." *Journal of Applied Social Psychology* 26, no. 22 (1996): 1985–2013.

Hall, Joshua M. "Philosophy of Dance and Disability." *Philosophy Compass* 13, no. 12 (2018): e12551.

Hancock, Black Hawk. "4. STEPPIN'OUT OF WHITENESS." In *American Allegory*, pp. 161–194. University of Chicago Press, 2013.

Harris, Cheryl I. "Whiteness as Property." *Harvard Law Review* 106 (1993): 1707–1791.

Harris, Lasana T., and Susan T. Fiske. "Dehumanizing the Lowest of the Low: Neuroimaging Responses to Extreme Out-Groups." *Psychological Science* 17, no. 10 (2006): 847–853.

Harris, Michael M., Filip Lievens, and Greet Van Hoye. "'I think they discriminated against me': Using Prototype Theory and Organizational Justice Theory for Understanding Perceived Discrimination in Selection and Promotion Situations." *International Journal of Selection and Assessment* 12, no. 1-2 (2004): 54–65.

Hayes, Cleveland, and Nicholas D. Hartlep, eds. *Unhooking from Whiteness: The Key to Dismantling Racism in the United States.* Springer Science & Business Media, 2013.

Holroyd, Jules, and Katherine Puddifoot. "6. Epistemic Injustice and Implicit Bias." *An Introduction to Implicit Bias: Knowledge, Justice, and the Social Mind*, 2020.

Holroyd, Jules, Robin Scaife, and Tom Stafford. "Responsibility for Implicit Bias." *Philosophy Compass* 12, no. 3 (2017): e12410.

Howard, Theresa Ruth. "Op-Ed: Why We Need to Confront Bias in Dance Criticism." *Dance Magazine,* August 3, 2017. https://www.dancemagazine.com/op-ed-we-need-to-confront-racial-and-cultural-biases-in-dance-criticism-2468342343.html. Accessed December 4, 2020.

Hudson, Sa-kiera Tiarra Jolynn, Mina Cikara, and Jim Sidanius. "Preference for Hierarchy Is Associated with Reduced Empathy and Increased Counter-Empathy Towards Others, Especially Out-Group Targets." *Journal of Experimental Social Psychology* 85 (2019): 103871.

"The Invention of Race." MPRNews.org. https://www.mprnews.org/story/2017/12/05/the_invention_of_race. Accessed April 29, 2018.

Isaac, Carol, Barbara Lee, and Molly Carnes. "Interventions That Affect Gender Bias in Hiring: A Systematic Review." *Academic Medicine: Journal of the Association of American Medical Colleges* 84, no. 10 (2009): 1440–1446.

Jackson, Philip Wesley. *Life in Classrooms.* Teachers College Press, 1990.

James, Robin. "Oppression, Privilege, & Aesthetics: The Use of the Aesthetic in Theories of Race, Gender, and Wexuality, and the Role of Race, Gender, and Sexuality in Philosophical Aesthetics." *Philosophy Compass* 8, no. 2 (2013): 101–116.

Johnson, Don Hanlon, ed. *Diverse Bodies, Diverse Practices: Toward an Inclusive Somatics.* North Atlantic Books, 2018.

Just Associates and We Rise. "Flower Power: Our Intersecting Identities." https://werise-toolkit.org. Accessed June 26, 2021.

Kant, Immanuel. *Observations on the Feeling of the Beautiful and Sublime.* University of California Press, 2003.

Kendi, Ibram X. *How to Be an Antiracist.* One World, 2019.

Kerr-Berry, Julie. "Counterstorytelling in Concert Dance History Pedagogy: Challenging the White Dancing Body." In *The Palgrave Handbook of Race and the Arts in Education,* pp. 137–155. Palgrave Macmillan, 2018.

Kerr-Berry, Julie, Ed.D. "Progress and Complacency: A 'Postracial' Dance in Higher Education?" *Journal of Dance Education,* 10:1 (2010), 3–5, DOI: 10.1080/15290824.2010.10387151. Accessed May 28, 2021.

Kolber, Jerry, and Bill Margol. *Brain Games.* Directed by Michael Simon. October 9, 2011. Los Angeles: National Geographic Channel, 2011.

Kuppers, Petra. "Accessible Education: Aesthetics, Bodies and Disability." *Research in Dance Education* 1, no. 2 (2000): 119–131.

Lakoff, George, and Mark Johnson. *Metaphors We Live by.* University of Chicago Press, 2008.

Lather, Patricia A., and Christine S. Smithies. *Troubling the Angels: Women Living with HIV/AIDS.* Westview Press, 1997.

Lepecki, André. *Of the Presence of the Body: Essays on Dance and Performance Theory.* Wesleyan University Press, 2004.

Lerman, Liz, and John Borstel. *Liz Lerman's Critical Response Process: A Method for Getting Useful Feedback on Anything You Make, from Dance to Dessert.* Liz Lerman Dance Exchange, 2003.

Levin, David Michael, ed. *Modernity and the Hegemony of Vision.* University of California Press, 1993.

Levinson, Justin D. "Forgotten Racial Equality: Implicit Bias, Decisionmaking, and Misremembering." *Duke LJ* 57 (2007): 345–424.

Lipsitz, George. "The Possessive Investment in Whiteness." *White Privilege: Essential Readings on the Other Side of Racism* 2 (2005): 67–90.

Macedonia, Manuela. "Embodied Learning: Why at School the Mind Needs the Body." *Frontiers in Psychology* 10 (2019): 2098.

Martin, Carol Lynn, and Diane Ruble. "Children's Search for Gender Cues: Cognitive Perspectives on Gender Development." *Current Directions in Psychological Science* 13, no. 2 (2004): 67–70.

Mason, Elinor. "Respecting Each Other and Taking Responsibility for Our Biases." *Social Dimensions of Moral Responsibility* (2018): 163–184.

McCarthy-Brown, Nyama. *Dance Pedagogy for a Diverse World: Culturally Relevant Teaching in Theory, Research and Practice.* McFarland, 2017.

Works Cited

McCarthy-Brown, Nyama. "Owners of Dance: How Dance Is Controlled and Whitewashed in the Teaching of Dance Forms." In *The Palgrave Handbook of Race and the Arts in Education*, pp. 469–487. Palgrave Macmillan, 2018.

Menakem, Resmaa. *My Grandmother's Hands: Racialized Rrauma and the Pathway to Mending Our Hearts and Bodies*. Central Recovery Press, 2017.

Mengel, Friederike, Jan Sauermann, and Ulf Zölitz. "Gender Bias in Teaching Evaluations." *Journal of the European Economic Association* 17, no. 2 (2019): 535–566.

Mills, Charles. "White Ignorance." *Race and Epistemologies of Ignorance* 247 (2007): 26–31.

Molden, Daniel C. "Understanding Priming Effects in Social Psychology: What Is 'Social Priming' and How Does It Occur?" *Social Cognition* 32, Supplement (2014): 1–11.

Monroe, Raquel L. "'I Don't Want to do African ... What About My Technique?': Transforming Dancing Places into Spaces in the Academy." *Journal of Pan African Studies* 4, no. 6 (2011): 38–55.

Montgomery, Mary Lynn, and Mary Jetter. "'I am from' Activity Guide: A Tool to Foster Student Interaction in the Classroom." Global Programs and Strategy Alliance at the University of Minnesota, 2016. https://global.umn.edu/icc/documents/I_Am_From_Faculty_Guide.pdf. Accessed May 8, 2021.

Moore, Carol-Lynne, and Kaoru Yamamoto. *Beyond Words: Movement Observation and Analysis*. Routledge, 2012.

Negowetti, Nicole. "Implicit Bias and the Legal Profession's 'Diversity Crisis': A Call for Self-Reflection." *Nevada Law Journal* 15 (2015): 431–460.

Nickerson, Raymond S. "Confirmation Bias: A Ubiquitous Phenomenon in Many Guises." *Review of General Psychology* 2, no. 2 (1998): 175–220.

Noble, Safiya Umoja. *Algorithms of Oppression: How Search Engines Reinforce Racism*. NYU Press, 2018.

O'Brien, Kerry S., John A. Hunter, and Mike Banks. "Implicit Anti-Fat Bias in Physical Educators: Physical Attributes, Ideology and Socialization." *International Journal of Obesity* 31, no. 2 (2007): 308–314.

O'Meara, KerryAnn, Dawn Culpepper, and Lindsey L. Templeton. "Nudging Toward Diversity: Applying Behavioral Design to Faculty Hiring." *Review of Educational Research* 90, no. 3 (2020): 311–348.

The Open Book Blog. Where Is the Diversity in Publishing? The 2019 Diversity Baseline Survey Results. https://blog.leeandlow.com. Accessed January 4, 2021.

Painter, Nell Irvin. *The History of White People*. W.W. Norton, 2010.

Payne, B. Keith, and Bertram Gawronski. "A History of Implicit Social Cognition: Where Is It Coming From? Where Is It Now? Where Is It Going?" *Handbook of Implicit Social Cognition: Measurement, Theory, and Applications* 1 (2010): 1–15.

Pierce, Edgar F., and Myra L. Daleng. "Distortion of Body Image Among Elite Female Dancers." *Perceptual and Motor Skills* 87, no. 3 (1998): 769–770.

Pinkus, Ari. "After the People of Color Conference, 10 Guideposts on the Path Toward Equity and Inclusion," National Assn. of Independent Schools People of Color Conference. Dec. 9, 2015, Tampa, FL. https://www.nais.org/learn/independent-ideas/december-2015/after-the-people-of-color-conference,-10-guidepost/.

Pinkus, Ari. "On Eve of the 28th Annual People of Color Conference, a Q&A with NAIS's Caroline Blackwell," National Assn. of Independent Schools People of Color Conference. Dec. 1, 2015, Tampa, FL. https://connect.nais.org/blogs/ari-pinkus/2015/12/01/on-eve-of-the-28th-annual-people-of-color-conference-a-qa-with-naiss-caroline-blackwell.

Preston-Dunlop, Valerie, and Ana Sanchez-Colberg. *Dance and the Performative: A Choreological Perspective—Laban and Beyond*. Verve Publishing, 2002.

"Project Implicit." https://implicit.harvard.edu/implicit/takeatest.html. Accessed April 29, 2018.

Rasmussen, Birgit Brander, Irene J. Nexica, Eric Klinenberg, and Matt Wray, ed. *The Making and Unmaking of Whiteness*. Duke University Press, 2001.

Relles, Stefani R. "A Call for Qualitative Methods in Action: Enlisting Positionality as an Equity Tool." *Intervention in School and Clinic* 51, no. 5 (2016): 312–317.

Richards, Thomas. *At Work with Grotowski on Physical Actions*. Routledge, 2003.

Sanchez, Jafeth E., and Bill Thornton. "Gender Issues in K-12 Educational Leadership." *Advancing Women in Leadership Journal* 30 (2010).
Schmidt, Sheri. "Cycle of Oppression." http://www.uas.alaska.edu/juneau/activities/safezone/docs/cycle_oppression.pdf. Accessed May 29, 2018.
Schupp, Karen. "Dance Competition Culture and Commercial Dance: Intertwined Aesthetics, Values, and Practices." *Journal of Dance Education* 19, no. 2 (2019): 58–67.
Schupp, Karen, and Nyama McCarthy-Brown. "Dancing with Diversity: Students' Perceptions of Diversity in Postsecondary Dance Programs" (2018).
Schwartz, Marlene B., Lenny R. Vartanian, Brian A. Nosek, and Kelly D. Brownell. "The Influence of One's Own Body Weight on Implicit and Explicit Anti-Fat Bias." *Obesity* 14, no. 3 (2006): 440–447.
Sechrist, Gretchen B., and Charles Stangor. "Perceived Consensus Influences Intergroup Behavior and Stereotype Accessibility." *Journal of Personality and Social Psychology* 80, no. 4 (2001): 645–654.
Sensoy, Özlem, and Robin DiAngelo. *Is Everyone Really Equal? An Introduction to Key Concepts in Social Justice Education*. Teachers College Press, 2012.
Shapiro, Sherry B. *Dance, Power, and Difference: Critical and Feminist Perspectives on Dance Education*. Human Kinetics, 1998.
Shotwell, Alexis. "Shame in Alterities: Adrian Piper, Intersubjectivity, and the Racial Formation of Identity." In *the Shock of the Other*, pp. 127–136. Brill, 2007.
Siegel, Marcia B. "Bridging the Critical Distance." *The Routledge Dance Studies Reader*, pp. 91–97. Routledge, 1998.
Singleton, Glenn E. *Courageous Conversations About Race: A Field Guide for Achieving Equity in Schools*. Corwin Press, 2014.
Sloss, Daniel, dir. *Daniel Sloss: X*. 2019; Sydney, AU: HBO Max, 2020, https://www.hbo.com/specials/daniel-sloss-x.
Smith, Phillip A. "Does Racism Exist in the Hiring and Promotion of K-12 School Administrators?" *Urban Education Research & Policy Annuals* 4, no. 1 (2016): 122–136.
Spears, Courtney Celeste. "How Dance Students Can Confront Racism and Implicit Bias in the Studio." *Dance Spirit*, June 10, 2020. https://www.dancespirit.com/students-confront-racism-2646167153.html. Accessed December 4, 2020.
Staats, Cheryl. "Understanding Implicit Bias: What Educators Should Know." *American Educator* 39, no. 4 (2015–2016): 29–33, 43.
Stinson, Susan W. "The Hidden Curriculum of Gender in Dance Education." *Journal of Dance Education* 5, no. 2 (2005): 51–57.
Storey, Valerie A., and Victor CX Wang. "Critical Friends Protocol: Andragogy and Learning in a Graduate Classroom." *Adult Learning* 28, no. 3 (2017): 107–114.
Sue, Derald Wing. *Microaggressions in Everyday Life: Race, Gender, and Sexual Orientation*. John Wiley & Sons, 2010.
Sue, Derald Wing, Christina M. Capodilupo, Gina C. Torino, Jennifer M. Bucceri, Aisha Holder, Kevin L. Nadal, and Marta Esquilin. "Racial Microaggressions in Everyday Life: Implications for Clinical Practice." *American Psychologist* 62, no. 4 (2007): 271–286.
Tajfel, H., and J.C. Turner. "The Social Identity Theory of Inter-Group Behavior." In S. Worchel and L.W. Austin LW, eds. *Psychology of Intergroup Relations*. Nelson-Hall, 1986.
Taylor, Charles. "The Politics of Recognition." *New Contexts of Canadian Criticism* 98 (1997): 25–73.
Tomiyama, A. Janet, Deborah Carr, Ellen M. Granberg, Brenda Major, Eric Robinson, Angelina R. Sutin, and Alexandra Brewis. "How and Why Weight Stigma Drives the Obesity 'Epidemic' and Harms Health." *BMC Medicine* 16, no. 1 (2018): 1–6.
Vai, Isabelle. Dance Data Project. July, 2020. https://www.dancedataproject.com/research/. Accessed April 23, 2020.
Vincent, Christian John-Devi. "Bridging the Gap: Between Commercial Dance and Dance in Higher Education." PhD diss., UC Irvine, 2015.
Wahl, Colleen. *Laban/Bartenieff Movement Studies: Contemporary Applications*. Human Kinetics, 2019.
Wernick, Laura J., Michael R. Woodford, and Alex Kulick. "LGBTQQ Youth Using Participatory Action Research and Theater to Effect Change: Moving Adult Decision-Makers

to Create Youth-Centered Change." *Journal of Community Practice* 22, no. 1–2 (2014): 47–66.

Whatley, Sarah. "The Spectacle of Difference: Dance and Disability on Screen." *The International Journal of Screendance* 1 (2010): 41–52.

Wilkerson, Isabel. *Caste: The Origins of Our Discontents*. Random House, 2020.

Williams, Riis. "Ballet Bias." *Real Change*. July 15, 2020. https://www.realchangenews.org/2020/07/15/ballet-bias. Accessed December 4, 2020.

Yakhlef, Ali. "The Corporeality of Practice-Based Learning." *Organization Studies* 31, no. 4 (2010): 409–430.

Yunkaporta, Tyson. *Sand Talk: How Indigenous Thinking Can Save the World*. Harper One, 2019.

Index

abled *see* nondisabled
adjudicators 44, 57–58, 146
aesthetics 7, 21, 43, 45, 48–49, 52, 57, 65, 67–68, 72, 81–82, 98, 106, 109, 118, 152, 155, 180, 190
African American *see* Black
Ahmed, Sara 132
appropriation 14, 34–35, 111–112
art 13, 49, 62, 67, 149, 172, 190
Avila, Homer 58

ballet 2–4, 13, 18, 21, 24, 36–40, 45, 50, 53, 56–58, 66–67, 70–71, 81, 125, 162, 181
Banaji, Mahzarin 18, 24, 62, 76, 108, 136, 138, 153
Bartenieff, Irmgard 2, 100, 145
Bell, Karine 135
bias: definition 11; explicit (definition) 10, 22; implicit (definition) 10, 19, 22; racial 1, 15–16, 25, 27, 69, 106, 136, 179, 180; testimonial (definition) 14
binary (thinking) 28, 42–43, 46–47, 51, 58–59
Black: African American 2–3, 16, 33, 46, 50, 55, 81; Black-bodied (visual marker) 23, 28, 68–69, 85–86, 92, 94, 105, 127; Black dance(r) 54, 71, 82, 92, 112, 178–179; black (skin color) 23, 104; race 1, 3, 5, 6, 15–17, 24–25, 32, 34–35, 40, 46–47, 60, 70, 73–74, 81, 135–136, 141, 153, 180–181; students 84, 90, 99–100, 126
Boal, Augusto 165
body prejudice 47, 98, 110, 127
brain-body 11–12, 20, 22, 25, 31–32, 45, 53, 88, 101, 124, 155, 163, 167–168
Bush, George W. 79–80

Cartesian 46, 134, 167
cata: qualitative 17, 67, 103, 137, 144, 150, 152, 165–166, 168, 170, 187; quantitative 6, 17, 24–25, 84, 91, 103, 123, 133, 137, 139, 142–143, 145, 165, 166
categorization 11–12, 18–19, 23, 25, 28, 37, 47–49, 53–55, 66–67, 70, 88–89, 96, 105–106, 113, 184
Chicago Steppers 37, 50
choreometrics 144–145
classical 45, 49, 52, 57, 71
Clemente, Karen 171, 78–80
cognitive busyness 80, 114–115
cognitive dissonance 24, 87, 116, 133–134, 138, 167, 191
Cohen, Stanley 70
commercial dance 37
competition 2, 55–57, 126, 146, 180
concert dance 24, 36–37, 39, 44, 49–50, 70, 105, 107, 113
confirmation bias 24–25, 69, 73
Copeland, Misty 71
Crenshaw, Kimberlé 59
Critical Friends Protocol 164
critical pedagogy 165
critical theory 7, 22, 103, 162
culture (definition) 22–24
cultural cloning 90, 139, 156

decision-making 16, 36, 47–48, 123–124, 140, 142, 147, 182–183, 186–187
demographics 15–16, 23, 83–84, 120, 137–141
denial 69–70
Descartes, René 89
DiAngelo, Robin 35, 41, 69, 74
disability 28–29, 40, 43, 51–52, 59, 70, 83, 123, 125, 136, 155, 162, 168–169, 172–173
discrimination 26, 35–36, 39, 44, 46, 51, 61–62, 78, 96, 122–123, 140, 144, 184
dominance 1, 14, 16, 23, 28, 33, 35, 37, 39–44, 52, 54–55, 57–61, 66–70, 72, 83, 85–86, 91–93, 99, 103–104, 106, 111, 126,

215

131–134, 145–146, 149, 155, 168–169, 186, 189

Eberhardt, Jennifer 74, 76, 126, 156–157
empathy 8, 72–77, 99, 118, 132, 146, 148, 162–163, 171, 175–176, 182, 192
entertainment 12, 48–49, 92
eugenics 73–74

Farnell, Brenda 102, 166–167
Fentroy, Chyrstyn Mariah 17
Fiske, Susan 76
funding (i.e. awards, funders, grants, scholarships) 18, 37, 39–40, 49–50, 60, 84, 92, 109

gender 1, 9, 22, 28–29, 31, 40, 43, 46–47, 58–59, 75, 83, 86, 90–91, 96, 116, 122, 125, 137–139, 173, 184–185
Gibbons, Elizabeth 158
Greenwald, Anthony G. 24, 76, 108, 136, 153

Hanstein, Penelope (Penny) 177, 184
Harris, Cheryl I. 15
Harris, Lasana 76
hegemony 49
hip hop 33–35, 37, 45–46, 66, 71, 181
Holroyd, Jules 111, 136
Howard, Theresa Ruth 18

identity 1–3, 9,-10, 16, 20, 24, 27–28, 31, 35, 40, 45, 52, 59, 65, 70–72, 78, 89–90, 92–93, 96, 104, 121, 123, 128, 134, 138–139, 144, 147, 155, 169, 171, 173–175, 185
implicit memory 12, 21, 48, 124
implicit social cognition (definition) 21
improvisation 33–34, 97, 109, 120, 130, 177
India 2–4, 9, 13, 103, 106, 111
internalized dominance 35
internalized oppression 34–35, 41, 139, 164
intersectionality 59

James, Robin 41, 43–45, 65, 67, 167

Kant, Immanuel 66
Kulick, Alex 165

Laban, Rudolf 100–102, 107
Laban Movement Analysis 43, 100–102, 104, 106–107, 109, 145, 171, 173–174, 181, 185
Lepecki, André 184
Levinson, Justin 14–15, 19, 25, 80, 91, 114
LGBTQ(Q) 83, 139, 141, 165
Lomax, Alan 145

Martin, Randy 184
McCarthy-Brown, Nyama 144
media 3, 32, 36, 39, 47, 54, 59–60, 65, 110–111, 113, 124, 153, 161
memory 4, 12, 21–23, 27, 35, 39, 41–43, 48, 54, 66, 79–81, 89–91, 99, 106, 114, 124–125, 154–155, 157, 170, 173, 185
Menakem, Resmaa 22–23, 67–68, 167
microaggression 47–48, 88, 92–93
Mills, Charles 70
mirror neurons 75–76
Monroe, Raquel 71
Moore, Carol-Lynne 11, 75–76, 82, 98, 107–108, 127–129, 145, 153, 162
movement analysis 98, 100–101, 103, 106–107, 111, 129, 163, 174
music 13, 33–35, 45, 105

National Association of Schools of Dance (NASD) 16
National Dance Education Organization 178
Natyashastra 103, 106
neutral(ity) 14, 103–108, 148–149, 163
North Carolina 2

objectivity 14–16, 19, 70, 83, 91, 97, 103, 107, 117, 122, 127, 129–130, 133, 142–144, 161, 166–167
oppression (definition) 31
organizational justice model 123–124, 140, 143–144

Paulay, Forrestine 145
Phillips-Fein, Jesse 92
Picasso, Pablo 127, 130
PK-12 schools 36–38, 45, 63, 94, 159, 172
(post)modern dance 2, 4, 9, 18, 33–40, 46, 50, 52–53, 57, 66–67, 70, 89, 97, 105–106, 118, 159, 178–179, 181
prejudice (definition) 35
priming 21, 27, 81, 124–125, 143, 152–153, 184
Primus, Pearl 112
private dance studios 36–37, 40, 60
prototype model 123, 140
Puddifoot, Katherine 111

Rancière, Jacques 65

St. Denis, Ruth 112
self-directed stigma *see* internalized oppression
Sensoy, Özlem 35, 188
Sloss, Daniel 12, 118
social dance 50, 66–67, 105
social dominance orientation (SDO) 52, 55, 75, 122, 128, 181

somatics 2, 8, 22, 67, 89, 133–135, 163–164, 167, 191
Spears, Courtney Celeste 18
stereotype 3, 24, 28, 32, 34–36, 46–48, 59, 75, 78, 88–89, 92, 94, 104, 114, 125–126, 129, 149, 152–154, 174, 182
Sue, Derald Wing 47

technique 13, 34, 46, 60, 71, 84, 98, 152–153, 159, 171, 180–182, 188
theater 5, 97, 161, 165

universal(ity) 13, 60, 63, 103–108, 125, 149, 163

vernacular dance *see* social dance

Weeks, Edisa 58
Wernick, Laura 165
Western dance forms 37, 72, 105, 107, 126
White savior 27, 63
Williams, Riis 18
Woodford, Michael R. 165

Yamamoto, Kaoru 11, 75–76, 82, 98, 107–108, 127–129, 145, 153, 162

www.ingramcontent.com/pod-product-compliance
Lightning Source LLC
Chambersburg PA
CBHW032042300426
44117CB00009B/1161